THE REPRODUCTIVE SYSTEM

When Womplers Walking Babies bite the dust (commercially speaking) the Wompler Toy Corporation decides to strike it rich at the expense of the US Government, putting in for a massive research grant to develop a self-reproducing machine. It's easy to get the grant, and not *so* difficult to make the machine. The trouble starts when the little grey boxes, feeding on any metal they can find and drinking from the power supplies, get out of hand.

JOHN SLADEK has long been recognized as a leading satirist whose brilliant inventiveness demolishes the institutions and conventions of 20th century life and literature. His novels and short story collections include *Tik-Tok*, *Roderick*, and *The Lunatics of Terra*. He lives in Minneapolis and *The Reproductive System* was his first novel.

GOLLANCZ CLASSIC SF

JOHN SLADEK

THE REPRODUCTIVE SYSTEM

VICTOR GOLLANCZ LTD
LONDON 1986

First published in Great Britain 1968
by Victor Gollancz Ltd,
14 Henrietta Street, London WC2E 8QJ

First published in Gollancz Paperbacks 1986

© John T. Sladek 1968

British Library Cataloguing in Publication Data
Sladek, John
    The reproductive system.
    I. Title
    813'.54[F]   PS3569.L25

ISBN 0-575-03851-9

Printed in Finland by Werner Söderström Oy

To P.Z.

DID YOU SEE HER IN "HEIDI"?

Suppose that it is once more 196–, that fateful year, and suppose that you are passing through Millford, Utah, that most fated of crossroads. Population, a battered, bird-spattered sign informs you, is "3810 And Still Growing! Home of Shelley B—"

Home of Shelley something, Millford lies about half-way between Las Vegas, Nevada, and the North American Air Defence Command (NORAD) buried deep in a Colorado mountain. The name "Millford" is honorific; there has never been a stream through this part of the desert, nor a mill, nor anything to grind in a mill. Perhaps it was named ironically, or wishfully. Founders of other desert towns have, after all, given them pretty names, hoping that (by sympathetic magic) pretty reality would follow.

Millford is not pretty, it is worn and warped. There is little to distinguish it from Eden Acres, Greenville or Paradise. Its feed store, like theirs, is checkered red and white. Along its main drag lurk old familiar faces: The Eateria; The Idle Hour; Marv's Eat-Gas; The Dew Drop Inn Motel.

You, the casual tourist—say you are an Air Force General from NORAD on his way to get a divorce—are more interested in your odometer than in that Coca-cola bottling plant or whatever it is over there on the right. You are barely conscious of an ugly factory of glazed brick, with a glass-block window on its rounded corner. "Wompler Toy Corporation. Makers of—"

The worn sign slides past you, lost forever. There is only one sign you are interested in: "Resume Speed". Ah, there it is. And there's another: "You are now leaving Millford, Utah, Home of Shelley Belle. Hurry Back!" Your foot comes down on the gas, hard. The rattle of tappets asks:

> Who the hell
> Is Shelley Belle?

You are irritated with Millford. You are annoyed with your own faulty memory. You are bored with all ugly little desert towns with their smug signs: "Biggest Little City in the Universe!" You are hot and bored and tired, and you exceed the speed limit a little, fleeing from the place where world history is being made ...

5

CHAPTER I

THE WOMPLERS AT WORK

"She was a phantom of delight
When first she gleamed upon my sight.
... And now I see with eye serene
The very pulse of the machine."

WORDSWORTH

"SORRY I'M LATE, gang." Louie Guthridge Wompler, vice-president in charge of public relations, bounced into the conference room on ripple-soled shoes. He smiled at the other three members of the board, but they seemed not to notice.

"Where were you?" asked the president, Grandison Wompler. His jowls shook with annoyance. "We've got important business to discuss."

"Sorry, Pop." Louie threw himself into a chair at the right hand of his father. "I was getting in some work on my lats. You know, *latissimus dorsi*? That's here." He pointed a thick finger at his own armpit.

"We're dissolving the company, son."

"You know, I'm getting some pretty clean definition—Dissolving the company! But why, Pop? Why?"

Grandison's gavel made a sound like a pistol shot. "Meeting to order," he rumbled.

"What's the scoop, Pop?" Louie persisted, and shone upon his father a winning, Harold Teen smile.

"Son," the old man began, then stopped. He was searching for a cliché that Louie could grasp. Though forty-one years old he did not seem, at times, far removed from adolescence. Now, as he toyed with a spring grip developer and a jar of SooperProteen tablets, Louie seemed even—his father frowned at the thought —even childish.

The two men did not look much like father and son. The president was tall, sunburnt and rangy, fleshing out slightly in his middle age to a dignified thickness. His face was heavy and serious, with a stern jaw and thick, dark brows. There were, however, laugh lines, and his black eyes were festooned with kindly wrinkles. With no grey in his hair, Grandison ("Granny") Wompler looked ten years younger than his sixty-five.

Louie, known by some as "Louie the Womp", was pale and porcine. He somehow managed to resemble a water-colour of his father, one which had been through the laundry. His blond, tentatively wavy hair, milk-coloured eyes and pastry-cook skin might have made him effete but for his immense bulk. There was something athletic in Louie's sagging shoulders and pyknik belly; he seemed a man who had been hit repeatedly in the face. His nose was flattened, and indeed all his features were a trifle smooth, a trifle melted.

He wore no tie, and beneath the white fabric of his shirt could be discerned the T-shirt legend: "SOOPERPROTEEN CLUB". His smile, as he waited for his father to go on, was as pure and meaningless as that of dentures in a glass, and as constant.

"Son, I don't know how I'm going to explain this to you—"

"Let me try, Granny." Gowan Dill, the joky ninety-year-old production manager, turned to Louie and said, "What your father wants to say is, we've hitched our wagon to a falling star."

"Summer slump, that's all it is," Louie whined, still smiling. "Sales gotta pick up by Christmas."

"We'll be *rooned* by Christmas!" snarled his father. "*Rooned!*"

"—summer slump, or—"

"No, son. The truth is, we're finished. No one wants Wompler's Walking Babies any more."

Grandison's gnarled hands trembled slightly as they lifted a doll from its tissue paper packing and placed it on its feet. It began to toddle along the polished surface of the table, mewing at every step. The president's jaw clenched with emotion. A kazoo in his head was faintly playing "The March of the Wooden Soldiers".

Hardly anyone knew what really happened to Shelley Belle. She had been put away in tissue paper, so to speak, with other, happier memories of the thirties (Al Jolson, Bank Nite movies, the Cord roadster, Paul Whiteman's orchestra), as though she were indeed a sunny, golden-haired doll. Just as no one wished to remember the real thirties (soup lines, bread lines, work lines), so no one wished to remember the real history of Shelley (grown, married, divorced, married, suicide attempt, bit parts in Alfred Hitchcock movies). She would always be as they first knew her, in 1935, tossing her curls and grinning impishly at W. C. Fields or Wallace Beery. All over America, housewives clutched their free dishes and gaped. As this five-year-old shrugged, tap-dancing her way through "The March of the Wooden Soldiers", they *tsked* in blank amazement. Wasn't she precious? Wasn't she the darlingest, sassiest, ittiest yummykins sweetheart, though? Wasn't she a living doll?

Doll. The word exploded in the brain of Grandison Wompler during a performance of *Heidi* at the Belmont Theatre. He had leaped up and begun cursing joyfully, until the manager, Ned Lambert, had been obliged to throw him out. Granny didn't mind. He didn't even mind missing the Spin-O-Cash. What were a hundred silver dollars to him? He was bursting with a million-dollar plan! He went straight home and wrote, in the centre of a sheet of paper: "DOLL = DOLLARS".

Why not make dolls of Shelley Belle right here in her home town, and why not distribute them all over the nation—the world? He would by God make a million and put Millford on the map at the same time.

There had been a few catches, as time went on. He had already got production started when a court order enjoined him from use of the name "Shelley Belle". But Grandison had established his market; he did not need her name any longer. Soon, Wompler's Walking Babies became famous in their own right, and his fortune was assured.

Even during the war he'd done well. The main plant had turned to making howitzer shells, while the seamstresses sewed canteen covers. The company had won two "E" awards. Louie had gone into the army and been decorated with the Quartermaster's Cross. It seems he had bought more canteen covers than any other quartermaster. Father and son had been sorry to see the enemy give up so easily.

In 1946 Wompler's Babies walked again, but not nearly so profitably. Sales kept slipping, slipping, as people forgot about the ageing, alcoholic Shelley Belle. Now, twenty years later, the factory had come to a stop. As Gowan Dill put it, with many winks and digs of his frail elbow, "Production has come to the end of the line, boys. The eye division is tight shut. Not a head rolling off the assembly line. We might just as well take the remainder of our dolls and—"

"Stuff them, I know," said Grandison wearily. "I know, I know, I know." He stared, bleary-eyed, at the doll walking away from him.

It had huge blue eyes and gold, stiff, sausage curls. It wore a

8

red-white-and-blue pleated dress with silver spangles, and a tiny pillbox hat. Its pink dimpled knees were barely visible between the silver fringe of the skirt and the thick white boots with silver tassels.

"Mew, mew, mew, mew, mew," it said.

"Looks swell to me, Pop," said Louie loyally. He had caught his fist inside the jar of SooperProteen tablets. It had not occurred to Louie not to reach into a jar with the spring grip developer in his hand. "I think it's a neat little product."

"But it isn't wanted, son. Little girls don't want Wompler's Walking Babies any more. They want Barby dolls. Dolls they can dress up in fashions." His voice grew thick with fury, and he flushed purple beneath his sunburn. "Dolls that can't walk a single step!"

"Gee, Pop, that's keen! Why don't *we* build a doll they can dress up?"

"Because we don't know the first thing about fashion, that's why. Mrs. Lumsey's seamstresses can't sew anything but spangles and pleats."

"And canteen covers," cracked Dill, shooting his cuffs.

No one was smiling. Grandison stared at the walking doll, looking as if he wanted to cry, but was just too strong. Louie was staring, mystified, at his entrapped hand. Moley, the chairman, was sliding down in his chair, preparing to sleep.

"Send this company to camp!" ventured Dill. No response. "Ah well," he sighed. "Let's put on our thinking caps."

The doll, still mewing, walked off the end of the table. There came the crack of a gutta percha face against the floor.

"The end of a great era," the president muttered hoarsely.

They thought. Louie had a hard time concentrating. He wanted to be outside, doing some road-work, or just getting a tan. He wanted to study up on his karate. He wanted to get home to see if that book had come in the mail: *Seventeen* New *Ways to Kill a Man with Your Bare Hands*. And the book on Sumo wrassling.

The trouble with books was, they didn't give a guy the *feel* of killing with his bare hands. That was the trouble with living in Millford, too. There was nowhere a guy could go to learn from an instructor. Louie wanted to learn all those Jap systems of self-defence. He wanted to learn how to kill a man with Zen—without even touching him, they say. Then there was Kabuki, and there was deadliest Origami. Man!

He continued staring out the window for inspiration, until a car, air-force blue, whizzed by. It reminded him of isometric exercises. Then, somewhere in Louie's rudimentary forebrain, a tiny circuit completed itself.

"I got it!" he shouted. "I got an idea!"

Dill groaned. "Not another idea," he said. "We haven't even finished paying for that coffee machine yet."

Louie's last brain-storm had been to sell the workers coffee from a machine he'd bought and installed in the cafeteria, at 25¢ a cup. To increase profits on the machine, he ran the grounds through again and again. The machine would thus, he reasoned, pay for itself. The workers agreed. The machine should pay for itself.

"No, this is a real keen idea. Listen. Why don't we get some money from the govermint?"

"Why don't we..." his father repeated uncomprehendingly.

"I think he has something, Granny!" shouted Dill. "Why *don't* we get some money from the government?"

"Oh, yes, indeed," said Moley, sitting up and opening his eyes a little. "He does have something. Why don't we—"

"Why don't we get some money from the govermint?" said Louie excitedly, and strained to complete the thought. His hand, encased in glass, waved impatiently. "From the govermint—for research!"

Bald heads nodded. "For research, yes!"

"But wouldn't we have to be making some product the government needs?" Grandison asked, puzzled. "Something vital to the defence of our nation? Something important to its welfare? The government doesn't just throw its money around, does it?"

When the others had finished laughing, Dill placed a bird-claw hand on Grandison's sleeve. "You're an old-fashioned, unpractical dreamer, Granny," he croaked, chuckling. "Maybe I am, too. We got to look to the boy here for *real* ideas. Times have changed since WPA, y'know. This here's the age of the astronaut. In the old days, I'll admit, you had to build a battleship or a municipal swimming pool—something useful. But tell me: practically speaking, of what use is it to have a man on the moon?"

"Well, I guess..."

"None! No *earthly* use at all," cackled Dill. "But seriously, the government spends millions, *zillions*, to put one man on the moon. On the other hand, if you have some real, some practical idea to sell them, forget it."

"That's right!" shouted Louie, jumping up and pacing about

the room. "Remember the time I tried to sell them my idea for invisible ink? Milk, it was, plain milk. Spies could write messages in it, like invisible ink. Then you heat it up and the writing appears, as if by magic. I wrote to the Pentagon, remember, Pop?" He threw himself into his chair again. "They never answered," he added, in a more subdued tone.

"The fact is," Dill went on, tapping his sere hand on the table, "if we can show the government a project that is utterly, hopelessly useless, they'll give us a grant for pure research."

"How do you know that?"

"I know it as sure as I know that the head of the Industrial Spending Committee is Senator Dill—my cousin, get it?"

Grandison was not yet used to the idea. "But—but what could we do research upon? We have no facilities."

"They provide all that stuff, don't worry," smiled Dill. "Concrete labs, bomb shelters, marine guards, you name it. All we have to do is figure out a project."

"How about a robot?" suggested Louie.

"No money in it," Dill snapped. "We need something which *sounds* easier, so that the rest of the committee can't object to it, but which is so hard in practice that we can spend years on it. Like a bigger, faster plane."

"How about a robot, though?" Louie put forth.

Ignoring the frantic waving of the jar under his nose, Moley said, "Now, why don't we build a machine that can reproduce itself? I was reading about an idea like that in *Life,* just the other day. A self-reproducing machine—sure sounds hard enough, don't it?"

"But what is it good for?" Grandison asked. "Besides making duplicates of itself, what is its function?"

"A robot," declared Louie softly, "could instruct me in hand-to-hand Kabuki."

"You still don't understand, Granny," Dill said, with a patronizing shake of his head. "It isn't good for anything. That's exactly what the government wants. What *we* want."

"I suppose you're right," said Grandison. He sighed. "It seems so dishonest."

"We'll be creating thousands of new jobs—for scientists, marine guards, government clerks who keep us on file."

"I know, I know, but will *we* make money?" the president snapped.

"Millions."

They voted at once. The vote was "aye" all around the table, to Louie.

"Aye, I guess," he muttered. "But hey, Pop, how about a robot, though? Huh, how about—"

Grandison reached over and cracked the jar with his gavel. The spring grip device leapt out, scattering glass and brown pills, and releasing the thick fingers of Louie the Womp from captivity.

"Motion carried."

CHAPTER II

ANOMALIES

"$u¢¢e$$!"
Sign on wall at Wompler Research Laboratories

"I, TOO, AM a failure," murmured Cal, staring at the jellyfish thing in the tank. It was supposed to be bright pink and right-side up. "This is the end for me too, old *Plagyodus*. I've ruined my last experiment."

He did not deem it necessary to add that it was his first experiment at Wompler Research, or that he had only been hired through the wonderful mistake of an IBM machine. The grey, deflated mass in the tank did not seem to be listening, anyway. A twisted rope of multicoloured wires rose from it to a panel of dials. The dials were all at zero.

Sighing, Cal began to write on the chart hanging next to the tank, "Biomech. arrgt. 173b aborted 1750 hours".

It was more than a job he would be losing; it was a chance to do work leading to a doctorate. *Everything I touch,* he thought, *turns to failure.* As if bearing out his words, the ballpoint pen ran dry.

Experimenting, he found that it would write on his hand perfectly, but not on the wall chart. He covered his palm with blue scrawls and trial signatures: "Calvin Codman Potter, Ph.D".

"It's the angle," said Hamuro Hita, the project statistician. "It won't feed ink uphill."

Cal blushed, corrected the angle of the pen and signed the chart. "Thanks. I guess I'm not very observant for an experimenter. In fact, I've just ruined this experiment. I suppose you won't be seeing much of me around here from now on."

"Oh, I don't think they'll can you for one mistake. What happened, anyway?" Hita spoke without pausing in his work, summing figures on an adding machine.

"I forgot to put the temperature control on automatic last night." Ripping loose the wires from their instruments, Cal hauled up the grey, dripping lump. "It—it poached, or something." Lifting the lid of a garbage can, he plumped in the jellyfish and stuffed in the bright stiff wires after it. Hita nodded at a chair by his desk, and Cal flopped into it.

"That's what'll happen to me, when they find out all about me," he said, indicating the garbage can. "The way they saw it, I was a bright, promising lad, having graduated at the top of my class at MIT. They expected me to set the world on fire. Whereas—"

"Whereas—?"

"I guess I'd rather not talk about it after all. Let's say I was hired by mistake, and I'm scared that any minute they'll realize it."

Hita nodded, and the two men lapsed into moody silence. Finishing his addition, the mathematician began cleaning his briar pipe with one blade of a pair of black-handled scissors. Cal stared about the lab, unable to conquer the feeling that he was saying goodbye to it all. Goodbye, QUIDNAC modular computer; goodbye, maze for phototropic "rats"; goodbye, solution in which grew a green crystalline tree, every branch of which formed part of an electronic circuit; goodbye, miniature automatic forge. He did not forget a goodbye to the main entrance, guarded by a stiff, humourless adolescent in the uniform of the Marine Corps.

"We're all flying under false colours here," said Hita, sliding a paperback book out of his desk drawer. "Do you know why the Womplers hired me? Because Louie wanted to learn Origami. The way he saw it, I'm Japanese, *ergo* ..."

"I don't believe it!"

"But you've only been here a week. You hardly know the Womplers, father and son. You haven't even met the project head, Dr. Smilax. I assume your main dealings have been with *them*."

"Meaning the Mackintosh brothers?"

Hita smiled. "Or as some of us call them, the brothers Frankenstein."

"But what were you telling me about Origami?"

"Officially, I'm a mathematician. In fact, my duties include teaching Louie Origami. I've had to study up on it myself, of course. Luckily, I found this book at the drugstore." He riffled the pages of the paperback. "It's a good job, all the same. I can make enough money at this to start my own statistical lab soon, and I only need to be silly for a half-hour a day."

"But how have you fooled them, if you don't even know—?"

"It's easy. You see, Louie thought Origami was a kind of Japanese self-defence. I've been able to make up my own rules, mostly, as we go along (I told him I was 'black scissors', and he was properly impressed).

"As for Grandison Wompler, he seems to think I ought to speak Spanish, for some reason. I rather like the two of them. There are even days when I can stand the brothers F. The only person around here who gives me the creeps is Dr. Smilax himself."

"Have you met him? What's he like?" asked Cal.

"No, I haven't met him, and neither has anyone else I know of, except the twins; that's the odd thing about him. No one even seems to know anything about him except that he's a surgeon and a biochemist. You'd think the head of a research team would at least want to meet his subordinates, but he's so inaccessible—"

Cal nudged him and pointed to the entrance, above which a red bulb had begun glowing. The marine guard drew his automatic and covered the two persons entering, until they showed him the red badges of Kurt and Karl Mackintosh.

Kurt skipped to get into step with his twin, and they strode on across the lab rapidly.

Their immense, bulging foreheads, exaggerated by advanced baldness and invisibly pale eyebrows, loomed over tiny, pouting faces to give them the look of kewpies or dimestore cherubs. They were plump and sexless creatures, these two, and it was hard to believe them the best cybernetics engineers this side of the Iron Curtain. The only features they possessed that were not of idiot quality were their eyes. Restless, flickering, intelligent, they were the colour of bluebottle flies.

The brothers flicked a glance at the empty tank, another at the chart, another at Cal.

"We expected more of an MIT valedictorian," Karl said nastily, as if speaking to his brother.

"That's right, Karl. He has not only ruined experiment 173b, but we have not had a single original idea from him, and he has not hypothesized a single biomechanical arrangement."

"True enough, Kurt." The brothers, perhaps because of their similarity, seemed to find it desirable to identify one another often. "True it is, Kurt. I begin to wonder if MIT's standards have not declined."

Hita cleared his throat. Steering themselves, as it were, by the clipboards under their arms, the two spun towards him. "But, gentlemen," he said, "Potter was just now discussing with me his new idea for a biomechanical arrangement. A sort of steel-shelled oyster, wasn't it, Cal?"

"Yes. A sort of—um—steel-shelled oyster. Yes. You see, it would have a number of advantages. Too numerous to mention."

"Such as—?" said the twins together.

"Well—instead of a pearl, it produces a ball-bearing. A slow way to make ball-bearings, admittedly, but then we're not really interested in the manufacture of—"

"I hope, Kurt, that he will follow out his line of inquiry," said Karl.

"And write a monograph," Kurt added. "But meanwhile we'll assign him to Project 32 as a special assistant. He can help wire up circuits, Karl."

Cal felt he had been both chastised and given a second chance. He was about to stammer out his thanks when the light above the door glowed a second time.

"Good evening!" boomed Grandison Wompler from the doorway. "Say, it's long after five, and we don't pay overtime, you know."

The Mackintosh twins drew themselves up slightly. Karl said, "Dedication to the human race cannot be curtailed by mere time."

"Our work goes on," his brother intoned, "day and night, committed ever to the achievement of peace in our time, final, eternal peace—"

"That's fine. But do you have to have all these lights on?" Grandison entered, waving aside the aimed pistol of the marine guard, and donned a white lab coat from a locker.

"Our newest project will consume immense quantities of power," Kurt informed him. "But it will benefit the human race immeasurably."

"Great. Good work, boys. But will it get me a new contract? Will it put Millford on the map? Will it make the government want to shower money on me?"

The twins looked at one another for a flickering second. "It will indeed," they chorused.

Louie stuck his head in the door and shouted to Hita, "Oh, there you are." He smiled and nodded at the marine guard, who was trying to decide whether or not to shoot him. "Hita, I'll meetcha in the gym, OK?" Hita smiled and nodded, and the ebullient intruder withdrew.

Grandison turned around and noticed the statistician. "Hi there, *amigo!*" he said grinning, and walked over to him, hand extended. Hita was the only member of the staff with whom Grandison ever shook hands. *"Como esta Usted?"*

16

"Muy bien," replied the Japanese, without enthusiasm.

"That's fine, fine. Now, if any of these fellows don't treat you right, you just come tell me, hear? I signed a government contract, and that means I got to give fair and equal employment to You Fellows. It don't matter what your race, creed, colour or religion is, you're all Americans!"

"But I'm not an American," Hita protested. Grandison affected not to hear him.

"Yes, I rebuilt this company from nothing, in less than a year —and I want to keep what we got. We got the finest cafeteria, the best coffee machines, the nicest bowling alleys and gym, the cleanest bomb shelters money can buy—and I want us to keep 'em. I want all you boys, black and white, to put your backs into it and really pull—for the company!"

"I'm sure we're all doing our best," said Hita, picking up a pair of scissors. "Well, I must go. *Adios.*"

"We, too, must leave, Kurt," said Karl. "We must confer with Dr. S. just now. Potter here can show you around the lab, Mr. Wompler." The brothers moved off, in lock-step.

"Say," said Grandison behind his hand. "I heard someone say their name was Frankenstein." His voice dropped to a confidential whisper and his face grew solemn. "They ain't—they ain't Jews, are they?"

"I believe they are Irish Protestants, sir," said Cal, trying to keep his face straight. "Their name is Mackintosh. Would you like to see the lab?"

"Yes, fine."

At each exhibit, Grandison would pause while Cal named the piece of equipment. Then he would repeat the name softly, with a kind of wonder, nod sagely, and move on. Cal was strongly reminded of the way some people look at modern art exhibitions, where the labels become more important to them than the objects. He found himself making up elaborate names.

"And this, you'll note, is the Mondriaan Modular Mnemonicon."

"—onicon, yes."

"And the Empyrean diffractosphere."

"—sphere. Mn. I see."

Nothing surprised Grandison, for he was looking at nothing. Cal became wilder. Pointing to Hita's desk, he said, "The chiarascuro thermocouple."

"Couple? Looks like only one, to me. Interesting, though."

A briar pipe became a "zygotic pipette", the glass ashtray a "Piltdown retort", and the lamp a "phase-conditioned Aeolian". Paperclips became "nuances".

"Nuances, I see. Very fine. What's that thing, now?" He pointed to an oscilloscope. Cal took a deep breath.

"Its full name," he said, "is the Praetorian eschatalogical morphomorphic tangram, Endymion-type, but we usually just call it a ramification."

The old man fixed him with a stern black eye. "Are you trying to be funny or something? I mean, I may not be a smart-aleck scientist, but I sure as hell know a television, when I see one."

Cal assured him it was not a television, and proved it by switching it on. "See," he said, pointing to a pattern of square waves, "there are the little anapests."

"I'll be damned! So they are."

Cal went on to show him a few revanchist doctrines before the president, satisfied, took his departure.

"Keep up the good work," he called out, "and take good care of the company equipment. Them ramifications don't grow on trees, y'know."

Cal began to chew his fingernails off, one by one, leaning against a lab table and dropping the parings in a Piltdown retort. *How long can I get away with this?* he wondered. *They still think I'm from MIT. And so I am. From Miami Institute of Technocracy.*

Miami Institute of Technocracy was the only school in the nation that gave a Bachelor of Applied Arts degree in biophysics. Cal had graduated in a class of four: Harry Stropp, Bachelor of Physical Education, Mary Junes, Home Economics Technician, Barthemo Beele, Associate of Journalism. Cal had headed the class.

I'll go confess to Dr. Smilax, he decided. *I can explain it was all a mistake.* He switched off the lights and left. The marine guard remained alone, standing at attention in the darkness.

Cal stopped at the hall bulletin board. A new notice had been posted, and now, stalling for time, he stopped to read it.

"PROJECT 32. Supervisors: DR. K. MACKINTOSH & DR. K. MACKINTOSH. Special Assistant: POTTER. Inspection will be 21 june 196–. At some time after this date, DR. A. CANDLEWOOD (Behavioural Psychol.) will join the staff."

Cal looked from the signature (impersonally mimeographed) to the door marked:

T. Smilax M.D.
NO UNAUTHORIZED PERSONNEL
THIS MEANS YOU
ABSOLUTELY RESTRICTED AREA

Changing his mind, Cal spun around and headed for the main door. As he passed the open window of the gymnasium building, he heard Hita shout, "Hai!" There was the sound of shearing paper.

CHAPTER III

A REPORT ON PROJECT 32

"He who understands me finally recognizes my propositions as senseless."

LUDWIG WITTGENSTEIN

TOP SECRET TOP SECRET TOP SECRET TOP SECRET

I. *The Purpose of Project 32*

Project 32 is the code name of a series of experiments undertaken at the Wompler Research Laboratory in Millford, Utah, in 196–. The purpose of Project 32 was to determine:

   (a) if it were possible to set into motion an autonomous, self-reproducing mechanism, a "Reproductive System", and

   (b) the military use, if any, of such a system.

II. *The Background of Project 32*

Prior to the initiation of this project, it was generally considered impracticable, if not impossible, to design and set into motion a system capable of self-support, learning, and reproduction. (a) Although computers had been programmed to perform simple analogies[1] or "learn", i.e., profit from their mistakes in straightforward games, they showed little promise as learning machines. And for a system to be autonomous, it must be able to discriminate portions of its environment, analogize from past experiences and profit from mistakes of a rather complex nature. (b) Although "autonomous" automated production lines already existed, they were at the mercy of their environments for power and materials. (c) Some computers had already been used to solve problems in circuitry, thus in effect "redesigning" themselves. But there re-

---

[1] Yet semantics vs. syntax arguments cast such doubts on these experiments as to make their results puzzling and amusing rather than significant. Thus while a computer saw the answer to "spear:?::narrow:arrow" was "pear", it could not see why "head:bed::?:chair" should be "back" and not "hair". Also a computer diagrammed the following sentence two ways: "She bears each cross patiently". "She" may be the subject and "bears" the verb; or "She bears" the subject and "cross" the verb.

mained what seemed an unbridgeable gap between these and a true self-reproducing machine.

III. *The Experiments*

Early experiments comprised attempts to construct living/non-living "symbioses": Inculcating in the nervous system of a coelentrate an electric motor circuit;[2] encasing oysters in shells of flexible steel;[3] equipping mice with electro-hydraulically-operated tails;[4] and many similar attempts, none satisfactory.

IV. *The Theory*

Out of these early experiments a modular of cellular system was conceived of, functioning somewhere between a polypidon and a highly structured society. Each cell should be:

(a) Organized along similar lines with its fellows, and equipped to recognize order and respond to it.

(b) Equipped to repair infracellular breakdowns, as far as possible, and to "eat" non-functional cells.

(c) Able to convert power and material from its environment into itself, and to construct new cells like itself from any surplus power and material, i.e., to reproduce.

(d) Able to prevent its own destruction by flight, by diversion of or neutralization of the destructive agent. E.g., if made of steel, it should (1) flee from sea-water contact; (2) paint itself to seal out sea-water; or (3) develop some chemical means to neutralize the corrosive action of sea-water.

No practical means were available to test or even construct a working model of this theoretical system, until the completion and adaptation of the QUIDNAC computer.

V. *The Quidnac*

The QUIDNAC, or Quantifiable Universal Integral DNA Computer, as originally designed by T. Smilax, had three qualities that recommended it to the project: (a) compact size; (b) a virtually infinitely-extensible memory; (c) suitability for learning complex analogic processes. In addition, T. Smilax was the head of Project 32.

[2] Failure due to unstable ambient temperatures, causing shock.
[3] Failure due to unforeseen corrosion, by sea-water, of steel.
[4] Successful, but of questionable military value. Results published separately as MIL-P-980089, PROSTHETIC TAILS.

VI. *General Principles of Construction of Cells*

Each cell may be considered in some respects an egg, having "yolk", "white" and "shell". In this simplified scheme:

(a) The "yolk" consisted of the QUIDNAC computer, along with various coupling and control devices to functions in the "white" and "shell".

(b) The "white" contained automatic production tools and storage facilities for raw materials, spare tools and parts, and power.

(c) The "shell" of metal armour contained means of locomotion, sensory devices, paint, simple extensors, and (though not in all cases) means of communication.

Within this framework many variations were constructed, differing in their means of locomotion, sensory devices, means of communication and production methods. It was expected that, in addition to variations proposed by the experimenter, others would be adapted or invented by the system itself.

* * *

"I just don't get it," said Cal, laying down his soldering gun. Though he spoke to Louie Wompler, all the army and navy technicians around them looked up, eager for a chance to stop and talk. Louie sat frowning at a folded piece of paper in his hand.

"Neither do I," he said. "Something wrong here. It's supposed to flap its wings when I do this, but look." He pulled at a flap, and the square of paper came unfolded. It was a magazine illustration of food.

"I mean I don't understand Dr. Smilax. What does he do all day, alone in there? He can't be still working on the QUIDNAC; I thought he finished with that long before he came here. Why do we never see him to talk to? What does he look like?"

Lance-corporal Martin looked up from a circuit diagram. "Are you kidding?" he said, pasting a Lucky in the corner of his wide, griping mouth. "I hear all kindsa crap about the Old Man." After looking around the room, he leaned closer to Cal. "I hear he carves up kittens on a big white table in there—just for kicks. I hear he's a junky. I hear he ain't no real doctor at all, just some bum chiropractor that saved a Senator's life once, so they give him this cushy job. I hear he just sits in there all day, sticking himself with dope. I hear—"

"Crap!" spat a navy technician whose rolled-up sleeves revealed tattoos of Walt Disney characters. "The real scuttlebutt is, he's a Rooshian. All that security stuff is to keep the other Rooshians from assassinating him. The real scuttlebutt is, he invented a way of putting monkey brains in the heads of little children."

A civilian technical writer spoke. He was the author of a famous military manual, *The Fork Lift Truck*. "I understand," he said carefully, "that Dr. S. used to be a famous surgeon. But he was operating on the President's mother and something went wrong. They hushed it up, of course, but he's been in semi-retirement ever since."

Others heard them and wandered over to join in.

"I hear the brothers Frankenstein was born joined at the head. He split 'em. But he gets fits, see, and tries to kill people—"

"—big abortion racket, remember? In all the papers—"

"They say he invented a cancer cure in Rooshia, but he was hit in the head, see, and lost his memory—"

"Devil's food cake," sighed Louie over the picture. He seemed oblivious of the discussion raging around him. "I'm not allowed to have any sweets while I'm in training for Origami."

"—and the ASPCA would raise holy hell if they found out what he was up to. So—"

Cal finished his work and stepped into the hall to get away from the babble of sensational theories about Smilax. The facts about the man behind that restricted door were nil. Yet why did all the rumours about him contain a strain of hideosity? Why was it no one saw him as a harmless old recluse? Why did every story include paradigms of cruelty, madness, meglomanic importance? It was almost as if . . . but no one could start such rumours about himself. Himself? For a moment Cal wondered if there really were such a person as "T. Smilax, M.D." Placing his ear to the restricted door, Cal listened.

There came to him a faint, high-pitched mechanical whine. It was the snarl of a thousand muted dental drills, humming into a thousand rotting teeth. It paused for a moment, and he heard another sound: The whimpering of a small dog in pain. Almost as soon as this began, the mechanical whine started up again, overriding it.

As Cal re-entered the lab, Karl said, "We were just looking for you."

"We're ready for a test," Kurt explained. They stood, clipboards at the ready, one each side of the lab table, while Cal made final adjustments and turned on the system.

It was an array of grey metal boxes, each about the size of a cigarette package, stacked loosely together in a cube about two feet high. When the toggle switch, prominent on the top of any one box was thrown, it sent out a tuned starting signal to the rest; they were switched off in the same way.

As soon as each box was activated, it began to roll about on the table on its little casters, avoiding collision with its fellows. When all the boxes were moving, they resembled a complicated Brownian movement on the dark surface of the table, as they explored every inch of it.

Kurt and Karl placed bits and scraps of metal on the table. The smaller bits were at once devoured by individual boxes, but the larger bars attracted the entire brood. The grey packages, now the size of king-size cigarette cases, swarmed over them like ants, gouging away with tiny cutters and torches—and growing fatter. It made Cal shiver to look at their orderly feeding.

"Has anyone a watch?" asked Karl, looking intently at the watch-chain across Hita's vest. The mathematician sighed.

"All right," he said, giving up his half-hunter. "But take care of it, please. It's an antique eight-day watch. Irreplaceable."

Karl dangled it on its chain above the table. The boxes began quavering, altering their random movements. They clustered beneath the watch. Karl swung it gently, and the grey brood responded, excitedly tracking its movements. They began to climb upon one another, to stack themselves in a swaying, rolling pyramid, reaching towards the shape of its metal body, the sound of its ticking heart. The grey pile began a sympathetic trembling.

Each time they would nearly reach the watch, Karl would raise it higher. His childlike face had a look of cruel, rapt concentration as he teased the pyramid. It grew taller and thinner. Cal could see lower boxes gripping one another with extensors to steady the pile. Karl raised the watch a third time, a fourth.

The top box, standing on edge, split like a tiny suitcase. Two thin rods slithered upwards.

"What are those? Look like car antennae," said Louie.

"Look out!" shouted Hita. "It's making a grab for it."

"No it isn't," Karl assured him. "Just watch this."

The two rods passed the half-hunter and moved a link or two up the chain. They paused. A group of boxes stopped "drinking" at the lab table's DC outlet and formed chain from it to the pyramid. There was a sudden flashing fizz of light and the watch fell; the tiny suitcase caught it, drew in its horns instantly and snapped shut.

"Hey! Give that back!" The mathematician caught up the offending box and shook it. He tried to pry it open, then shook it again.

"Ouch!" Suddenly the box clattered to the table, where it scooted about madly and was soon lost among its kind. There was a drop of blood on the end of Hita's finger. "Bit me!" he exclaimed, incredulous.

"Yes." Kurt nodded enthusiastically. "You've got to expect it to fight back. You were threatening it."

"Yes, it was only defending its property," Karl added.

"*It's* property!" Hita looked from one of the twins to the other. They wore pleased smiles, like those of indulgent parents. Without another word, the mathematician stalked out of the laboratory.

"Let's see what it will do with this," chorused the brothers. They wheeled over the oscilloscope on its stand and jammed it against the table. The grey creatures took notice of it at once. They now varied in size, from those which had scarcely grown at all to those which had swollen to the size of small tool boxes. None had so far reproduced.

Now they swarmed around the oscilloscope and began to pile up against the side of it. From the top box a tiny screwdriver emerged to probe the cabinet. Finding a louvre, it pried. The shaft broke. There was a muffled click and its stump retracted.

"Watch," Karl cautioned.

Smoke rose from the tool box, and there came a sound of loud, rapid hammering. A moment later a large screwdriver blade, still glowing, appeared. By main force it pried open the cabinet of the oscilloscope, bending back the steel cover to open a fist-sized hole. From another box came a pair of pliers. They entered the oscilloscope cabinet and began to rummage hastily inside. There came the tinkle of broken glass from time to time. At regular intervals, the pliers emerged, bearing booty: a broken tube, a two-inch hank of wire, half a resistor or a glass shard. On these, the tool box fed greedily.

"Hey!" said Louie, coming awake to what was happening. "You better not let Pop see that."

It was too late. At the same time, Grandison put his head in the door. "See what?" He saw the tool box come up with a hank of transistors which it gobbled like succulent grapes. "What the hell is going on here?" Glowering at Cal, he shouted, "It ain't two weeks since I told you to take care of the equipment. What the hell do you mean, destroying my property like that?"

Cal moved to shut off the system, but Kurt laid a restraining hand on his arm. "No," he said. "It is making mistakes, but it will learn. We're having an inspection next week by General Grawk of the Air Force. Let it go until then. We'll give it a corner of the lab of its own, to grow in." Turning to the company president he added, "Don't worry, sir. This system will make the company billions for every dollar it costs."

"Well, that's a relief." Grandison's expression altered. "I got some bad news, though. Hita just died in the infirmary."

Cal stared. *"What did you say?"*

"Hita. The statistics man. Just died of snakebite."

With a small thunderclap, the cathode-ray tube collapsed. The tool boxes continued to browse quietly.

"Poor ramification," Cal murmured, shuddering. "Poor little anapests."

CHAPTER IV

THE INSPECTOR GENERAL

" 'Es ist ein eigentümlicher Apparat,' sagte der Offizier."
KAFKA

BY THREE O'CLOCK on the afternoon of the inspection, almost the entire staff of Wompler Research Laboratories had assembled on the lawn, wearing clean lab coats. They stood in serried ranks, so perfectly still that the loudest sound was the faint susurrus of the lawn sprinklers. At the fore, faces uplifted to the sun, stood Grandison and Louie, wearing lab coats especially designed for the occasion by Mrs. Lumsey.

At precisely three o'clock, a silver helicopter descended from the sun. Its terrific downdraft ruffled the American flag on the flagpole and the two "E" pennants below it. It stirred slightly the silver fringe on the pleated lab coats of the two Womplers. The helicopter settled in the lush carpet of green. A silver door swung open.

General Grawk emerged amid a cloud of beautiful women. Actually there were only four redheaded women, each very like the other three, that is, tall, good-looking, and possessed of curves even Air Force tailoring could not disguise as angles. Here were four sane, attractive WAF officers bustling about to adjust his ribbons, straighten his ties, hand him his cap and relight his black stump of a cigar—bathing, in short, in an ambience of lovely femininity—

The ugliest man within a thousand miles.

Imagine a face as red and furious as that of a newborn child. Imagine sparse black hair like broken quills, lying this way and that around a bald spot the colour of a baboon's bum. Imagine the nose of a Pekinese but the upper lip of Peking man, and imagine moreover the former permanently wrinkled with disgust and the latter drawn back in a set sneer from yellow, crooked teeth. Add boiled, bulging eyes, an underslung jaw that needed a shave the day it was created, and the neck of a particularly obese walrus, complete with three folds of fat in back. Got all that? Now add black clots of eyebrow and asymmetric lumps

27

as desired, set it all on a stumpy, strutting figure in uniform, and top it off—as Grawk now did—with a tall, tall cap loaded with silver foliage.

Putting on his cap increased Grawk's height to about five feet. He spat out the cigar and looked around, arms akimbo.

"So this," he said, "is the great Wompler Research Laboratory, is it?"

"Yes indeed. I'm Grandison Wompler and this is my son, Louie. Louie, say hello to General Grawk."

"Hi!" shouted Louie.

The general squinted the Womplers over, ignoring no detail but their proffered hands. "Cute little outfits you got there," he said, jabbing a finger at their silver fringe. "Who's your dress-maker?" Then to one of the WAF's, "Make a note of it, Meg. First of all, they got cruddy security. Nobody asked to see my ID card. I coulda been a Russky spy, for chrissake. Second, I think the two top boys are fruits. Father and son, my eye! And all dressed up in Mother's clothes, I guess, eh?"

Louie's grin wavered, disappeared. "Now wait a minute," he said. "Whose mother? Now just wait a minute." His immense pudgy hands became fists.

"Like to lose your old man a couple million in government con-tracts?" shrilled the general. "Like to fix it so you're out of government work for good? Well, just lay a mitt on me, Junior. Go ahead, hit me!"

Grandison managed to keep his son from complying. Grawk smirked slightly, stretched out the folds of fat in his neck, and peered around him. "Are we gonna stand out here all day?"

The entire ménage fell in behind Kurt and Karl, who guided the general to the outer door of the lab building. To Grawk's fresh indignation, a marine guard insisted on seeing his ID card.

"Great," he said, producing it. "Just great. This guy *can't see* I'm wearing the uniform of a general in the US Air Force. He has to *make sure*. Just swell. Oh, I can see this is a well-run place all right."

They moved on inside.

"Which one of you ginks is Smilax, head-of-project? You?" he asked Karl, who shook his head.

"He sends his regrets," Karl said. "He's unable to meet you in person."

"What do you mean, 'unable'? Where is he?"

"In his office." The twins pointed out the office door.

A bitter smile rippled over the simian lip. "I get it. I'm not important enough for him to get up off his bacon and come out to meet, is that it? A mere four-star general is nothing, huh? I guess he only talks to the Joint Chiefs of Staff or something."

As the twins made no reply to this, the general stepped to the office door and tried it. It was locked. Lifting a set of knuckles designed to be walked upon, he rapped smartly on the RESTRICTED AREA sign.

A nearby door opened, and a marine guard, bearing a submachine gun, stepped out.

"I'm afraid you can't go in there, general," he said. "'NO UN-AUTHORIZED PERSONNEL. THIS MEANS YOU'," he quoted from the quite legible sign.

"What the hell do you mean? I got a top secret clearance. I'm supposed to be inspecting this plant. If I ain't authorized, who is? What the christ is going on here, anyway? Smilax, you come out of there!" He rattled the knob and pounded on the door until the guard trained his gun on him and waved him away.

"Look," Grawk said to him, a more conciliatory note creeping into his voice, "I come seven hundred miles in that hot, stuffy helicopter to inspect Smilax's project. You mean to tell me this freak can't even come out of his office to talk to me?"

"I'm afraid not, general. Dr. Smilax comes and goes at his pleasure," said the marine tersely. "If you want to contact him, you'd better forward your message to the Joint Chiefs of Staff."

"———" said the general. That is, he opened his mouth but no sound came forth. Purple veins began to writhe in his face, and his boiled eyes bulged.

Then he turned on his heel, emitting at the same time a short, hysterical laugh. "All right," he said. "Let's see this so-called project, and get it over with."

In one corner of the lab a considerable space had been cleared. A bulky object roughly the size of an automobile here lay shrouded in a drop cloth. Now the Mackintosh brothers moved in to lift the cloth, folding it rapidly and expertly into a cocked hat.

"What's all this?" said the general, waving at the pile of large grey boxes thus revealed. They lay on three lab tables, quivering, turning slightly on their hidden wheels as they sensed movement about them.

"It is a self-reproducing machine," the twins announced. "A Reproductive System."

"Yeah? Ugly, ain't it?"

During the week, they explained, the boxes had devoured over a ton of scrap metal, as well as a dozen oscilloscopes with attached signal generators, thirty-odd test sets, desk calculators both mechanical and electronic, a pair of scissors, an uncountable number of bottle caps, paper clips, coffee spoons and staples (for the lab and office staff liked feeding their new pet), dozens of surplus walky-talky storage batteries and a small gasoline-driven generator.

The cells had multiplied—better than doubled their original number—and had grown to various sizes, ranging from shoeboxes and attaché cases to steamer trunk proportions. They now reproduced constantly but slowly, in various fashions. One steamer trunk emitted, every five or ten minutes, a pair of tiny boxes the size of 3×5 card files. Another box, of extraordinary length, seemed to be slowly sawing itself in half.

General Grawk remained unimpressed. "What does it do for an encore?" he growled.

"I don't know much about this stuff myself," Gandison candidly admitted. "I leave all the heavy think-work to my boys here, Kurt, Karl and Cal. They know all about Endymions and revanchist doctrines, all that stuff."

With savage glee, the general spoke to one of his WAF's. "Amy, make a note. I think this one is a commy," he spat with disgust, "as well as a fairy."

"Let me hit him, Pop!" bawled Louie. "Let me use Origami on him."

Kurt and Karl went on explaining the system, as though they had not been interrupted.

"It is 'ergetropic'," Karl explained. "That is, it can seek and use nearly any kind of power." He gestured to his brother as one vaudeville partner to another.

"It is metallotropic," Kurt added. "Some cells are oriented more towards metal, some towards energy. May we demonstrate?"

The twins each picked up one box gently. They were the size of fat attaché cases. "This is a power-seeking cell," Karl explained. "That one is metal-seeking."

The wheels of the two machines whined as they set them on the floor. One spun around and headed straight for the light socket. The other dashed about the room, sampling the legs of metal furniture, pausing to nibble at the corner of a filing cabinet. Cal shooed it away and it scooted behind a lab table, out of his reach. Between the table and the wall, he could see the box working its way along towards the far corner, towards the oyster tank.

"Kinda cute at that," said the general.

One of its legs eaten through, the oyster tank collapsed. As water from it spread across the flooor, the fat box outran it, heading for the door. It carried a metal wastebasket, holding it aloft in crab-claws, a hard-won trophy.

"Stop it!" Cal shouted. The general began to laugh.

"Halt!" shouted the marine guard. He fired a warning shot but the attaché case kept coming. He lowered his gun and fired direc-tly at the little box. Bullets rang on the wastebasket. The marine emptied his gun, just as the box dashed between his polished boots and out of the door.

"All you had to do," said Karl, "was pick it up."

The general leaned on the table, doubled up with coarse laugh-ter. The twins and Cal were trying to trap the other box. Excited by the gun-flashes, it scooted in circles all over the room.

"I'll be goddamned," the general kept saying. "Funniest thing I seen since the war." His weight was tipping the table, and as the boxes rushed towards him it tipped even further.

Cal cornered the energy-seeking box and bent to turn it off. He saw that the toggle switch had been damaged, apparently by a welding arc. It was a fused lump of metal on top of the box. Some-thing else occurred to him then: there had been a lot of cells running around on the table with broken or missing switches. Odd. He would have to ask someone about that.

But just now there was nothing to do but pick this one up off the floor. Cal was frightened of it, but he was even more fright-ened of letting it go free.

"Careful!" someone shouted. "You're standing in brine!"

"Oh, don't worry," said Cal. He looked up to see the table overturn on General Grawk, the boxes sliding off...

But then the scene froze, like a film hung up in the projector. And, like a stuck film, everything shrivelled and vanished, leaving only bright white emptiness.

CHAPTER V

M.I.T.

"O goodly usage of those ancient times,
In which the sword was servant unto right."
SPENSER

CAL WAS BROUGHT up on a farm in Minnesota. His father Codman Codman Potter, was taciturn, even for a farmer. In fact, Cal could only recall his father's speaking to him twice in all his life. Codman seemed a bottomless reservoir of wisdom; whenever he spoke, the family went into a panic.

The awful voice first sounded when Cal was eight. His mother had given him a book of Aesop's fables, and one evening he lay on the living room floor, reading of the frogs who wanted a king. His father looked at him and said loudly:

"There's plenty of things you don't learn from books. Books only ruin your eyes. It's life that's important, not god damned books!"

Alarmed, Cal's mother took the book from him and burned it. He never dreamed of objecting. From then on, he merely skimmed his lessons and school, and avoided bringing home any of the hated books. At home his only lapse was glancing at the back of the cereal box: "Niacin, Thiamine, Riboflavin..." Surely, he reasoned, it was all right to read, as long as he did not understand.

This idea of reading only the unreadable stayed with him until he asked his father for permission to study Latin and Greek.

"What? If you want to go to college at all, you'll by god become an engineer. Or else I'll Latin you, god damn it!"

Cal went off to the Miami Institute of Technocracy, then, to become an engineer. At the station, Codman nodded goodbye.

MIT was small. There were just twenty students and one professor altogether, and in Cal's class there were but three other students. The entire school occupied one large room above a dry-cleaning plant. In after years, Cal would always associate the smell of chemicals and the hiss of steam with Dr. Elwood Trivian.

"You have an interest in the inimicable classics? I laud that, young man. We have, alack, no time to teach them here. They are, you cogitate, useless. I must deplore you to study science, and science alone.

"I had a thorough grinding in the classics myself, and am today but a humble pedagod. Why, I earn less here in an entire year than I would in a single week on the railroad, steering a train! And that takes no learning at all!"

Half-way through his course, Cal switched his major from Engrg. Arts to Biophys. Arts. He wrote his father explaining that this had more to do with life. In a sense, he was telling the truth, for it enabled him to sit next to Mary Junes, whom he loved.

Mary did not love him back; she was not likely to love him; she did not even know his name. She seemed to love Harry Stropp, their tall, thickset, swart classmate, who majored in Phys. Ed.

She was a short, chunky, tough-looking girl with a great gob of yellow hair like dirty cotton. As everyday attire she wore borrowed sweatshirts, mixed and matched with dungarees and borrowed sweatpants. She seemed addicted to black cough drops. Her breath smelt of menthol, her hands were always sticky, and her wide, sluttish mouth was stained black. Cal dreamed of pasting a kiss on those gummy lips.

He schemed to sit next to her in every class: Current events (where Dr. Trivian read his morning paper aloud), Phonics Praxis and Appreciation of Thermodynamics. Still, her nights were spent with Harry.

Barthemo Beele, the fourth member of the class and a Journalism student, published the mimeo school paper, *The MIT Worker's Torch*. He bitterly complained of seeing Mary and Harry kiss in public, in editorials headed: "Is Decency Finished?"

One day Harry came down with a cold. After struggling through morning classes, he gave up and went home. Mary clicked a black cough drop deliciously, and winked at Cal. "What's your name?"

Harry arose from his sickbed in a week, to find he'd lost his girl to Cal.

"I don't care," he'd say, flexing his big arm and studying it. "She's not the only pebble on the beach. There are plenty of other fish in the sea." He remained an absolute recluse, going swimming and fishing alone, and doing lots of roadwork on the roof above the schoolroom. Cal felt terribly guilty every time he heard the sound of giant, sad tennis shoes on the roof, running tirelessly.

The MIT Worker's Torch named Cal valedictorian of the class. On the same day, it announced the engagement of Miss Mary Junes to Barthemo Beele.

"When did this happen?" Cal asked her, holding up the mimeo sheet in a trembling hand.

"Oh, you know that night last week, when you had to study?"

"But—*engaged*?"

"Yup. Right after graduation, me and Barty are going to live somewheres out West, where he's got a swell job as a editor already. Isn't that great?"

Great. The next few days Cal knew not what he did. He wept unashamedly, tore up all her notes ("Can I borrow your sweatshirt, darling? Thanx, M."), and took long walks, at times avoiding all meaningful places, at times haunting them. He began to feel he might become a dedicated scientist, a seeker after truth.

Most of the hundred foundations, academies and labs to which he applied for a research grant replied that they had no need for holders of the rather special degree, Bachelor of Biophysics Arts. The Wompler Research Laboratory, however, sent a letter expressing interest and an IBM card to fill out and return. In the tiny box on the card where he was to write the name of his school, there was only room for the abbreviation "MIT". He was hired by return mail.

The MIT Worker's Torch kept up its morality campaign (now directed against its editor and his fiancée) to the last day. Dr. Trivian gave a stirring Commencement speech to his four new graduates, though most of it was drowned out by the hiss of steam from below, where the shirts lived.

* * *

"Oh, don't worry," Cal said. It seemed to him that he was still trying to pick up the runaway cell, but bright white clouds kept getting in his way. Steam?

All at once he realized the clouds were real; he was looking at the sky. He rolled over and sat up, hands buried in cool grass.

A file drawer marked "Secret" scooted past, pursued by a mob of people in white coats. "Stop it! Catch it!"

How odd, he thought with a tolerant smile. Chasing file drawers. He began to walk around the building. Other boxes, made of garbage cans, cabinets, bent signs, swarmed over the green, pursuing and pursued by human figures. Near the fence a group of marines had set up a light machine gun. Now they were defend-

34

ing it desperately against the slow, blunt, methodical attacks of a kiln and a small safe, in tandem. Finally a fork-lift truck rushed in, seized the gun and apparently digested it.

Chuckling, Cal strode around another corner of the building. The helicopter lay on its side as the swarming boxes picked it clean. It was beginning to look like the skeleton of a beached whale.

The general was no longer laughing; he was screaming at the twin brothers, "Somebody is gonna have to pay for this! That is government property your toy is tearing up!"

"Government property hell!" Grandison roared. "That gizmo is tearing up *my* property! If you can't shut it off—"

"Mr. Wompler, General Grawk," said Karl solemnly, "there seems to be no safe way to shut it off—without jeopardizing the whole experiment, that is. We simply cannot permit it."

Grandison caught sight of Cal. "So you finally came to, eh?" he said. "Just in time, too. I guess one of them Endymions musta give you a little electric *shot*, eh boy? Well, I hope you can shut that thing off—Kurt and Karl here are chicken."

"There should be nothing easier than shutting it off," Cal said, "Every cell is equipped with a sympathetic, tuned switch that—"

"Not any more," said Karl with a condescending smile. "That was last week. The more sophisticated mutations of the system have shed that apparatus long ago."

"Well then, I'll shut off the ones that haven't, and we'll smash the rest."

"No, you don't!" Kurt said, bridling. "If you go in that lab and tamper, you're fired!"

Grandison wavered, less sure of himself now. "Maybe you shouldn't—"

"I'm not worried about protecting property," said Cal quietly. "I'm worried about protecting a few lives. None of you seem to realize how dangerous this thing is."

"What are a few lives, in comparison to—" Karl began, but Cal did not stay around to listen. He dashed around the corner to the main entrance and back to the lab.

It was scarcely recognizable. Larger and larger cells had formed, some viable, some not, which forced themselves into the corners of the room and ate away at the very structure of the building. Festoons of insulation hung above, where once there had been a fluorescent lighting system. Now the lamps and conduit were gone, and the very copper wires stripped from their insulation, which hung like abandoned snakeskins. There was not a scrap of metal in the room which had not been made into something else. Steel partitions, cabinets, desks had all been melted, running together in fantastic shapes.

There was a solid barrier before him, waist-high, of dead or dying cells welded together as dead polyps are clustered to make coral. He began to climb over them, looking for one with an intact toggle switch.

He found one, and threw it. The system shut off slowly, in stages. Cal heard the muffled whine of slowing dynamos in the basement, the dying fall of gears.

In the queer, sudden silence, he made his way out to the sunlight once more.

With the exception of a group of Marines, who were beating to death a small suitcase, the people who had been running madly about before were now still, scattered like groups of statuary on the lawn. The statues were all looking at Cal.

Grandison Wompler finally moved, shaking his head sadly. "I never thought you'd do a thing like that to me," he said. "Why, boy, why? I took you right out of school, I gave you the best opportunity a young man ever had to make something out of hisself, and here you stab me in the back, first chance you get."

"But—"

"Oh, don't try to worm your way out of it. I got the whole story from them Frankenstein fellows. You just turned a billion-dollar machine into a great big pile of junk."

"That's right," Karl said nodding emphatically. "You realize that shutting off the Reproductive System completely inactivated the QUIDNAC memory?"

"But it was running berserk!" Cal cried. "It's already killed one man. It might have—"

"Oh, it's easy for *you* to say what might have been," Grandison thundered.

"Don't, Pop." Louie laid a hand on his father's shoulder. "Don't get yourself worked up over *him*. He ain't worth it." He led his father away. Grandison's shoulders seemed to sag more with every step he took.

"Yas, a complete security blackout, button it up tight," said Grawk into a field telephone. He hung up and turned to face Cal. "Well, boys," he said to the Mackintosh brothers, "what do we do with this one? Shoot him? (We can do it legal, you know. Caught in an act of sabotage, etc. etc.)"

36

A kindly-looking middle-aged man in rimless glasses wandered near, and seemed to take an interest in the proceedings.

"No need to trouble," said Kurt, grinning. "He's harmless—now—and I'm sure by the time Senator Moley's committee get through with him—if you get my meaning?"

"Meanwhile, you're fired," said Karl brusquely. "Better get going before we have you arrested for trespassing, eh?"

Grawk laughed at Cal's look of consternation.

"Don't bother turning in your lab coat," Kurt said. "Or your pocket slide rule. Keep them. Just go."

"Has everyone lost their minds? I've just saved your lives, maybe, and you act like I'm Benedict Arnold. You, sir," he said, appealing to the kind-looking stranger. "Tell me, do I look like a traitor? Do you think my shutting off this damned machine is such a crime?"

The man smiled apologetically. "I'm afraid I'm really too prejudiced in the matter to be of much help," he said, and gave a small cough. "You see, I'm Smilax, and it's my machine you've just put to death."

There seemed nothing to do but go. As Cal walked away, he could hear the general talking about him in a very loud voice.

"There goes a helluva rotten bastard, if you ask me. A guy that would sell out his country like that—well, it's just lucky for him I ain't armed. Because if I was armed—" Grawk lowered his voice and added something Cal couldn't hear. Whatever it was, it made the four WAF's laugh very hard indeed.

He had lost his job, disgraced himself, submitted even to the flaying knives of pretty women's scorn. Cal was in no condition to do anything like rational thinking. For if he had been, there was one question he surely would have asked himself:

How was it a system as intelligent, as adaptable, as clever at self-protection as this one was supposed to be had given up almost without a fight?

CHAPTER VI

THE BOXES THAT ATE ALTOONA

*"I have taught my gears to talk
Nicky-nicky Poop, tic-toc."*

Louis Sacchetti (attrib.)

"Of Altoona, Nevada, lying quite near Parsnip Peak (8,905 ft.) and not far from Railroad Valley, where no railroads run, I sing," wrote Mary Junes Beele on her husband's L. Ç. Smith typewriter. Below it, she typed asterisks: a row of posies. The swollen belly of her thumb pressed the space bar.

From the next room came the clanking of a hand press. Editor Barthemo Beele was running off the second edition of the *Altoona Weekly Truth. His hand,* she thought, *that rocks the cradle ...* Mary cursed the paper and she cursed the paper's editor, her husband of one week.

The keys of the typewriter, she saw, were like black cough drops. Black cough drops were not to be had in Altoona. One of the typewriter's keys had broken one of Mary's nails. She began to chew it off, cursing everything she could think of—especially cursing Altoona. If that sailor did not take her away soon, she was going to die of this town. As she bit into another nail spitefully, contrary Mary cursed her rotten luck.

Altoona, too, had an unlucky history. In 1903, it had been the sole supplier of reuttite to the entire Western Hemisphere. Reuttite was of course that metal which made the best, most brilliant, longest-lasting gas mantles. There was no other known use for reuttite.

On Park Avenue in Altoona, the magnates of four different railroads had made their homes beside those of dozens of mine-owners and speculators. They'd built great white carpentered castles, gothic dreams in scrollwork and gingerbread, with bow windows, mullions, heart-shaped arches, wandering ivy and brave towers. The earth was shot through with old mine tunnels, so that now most of these heavy homes had sunk into it. Park Avenue was mainly a row of rusty fences and weedy lots. Occasionally one might glimpse through the hollyhocks a tower, its conical hat askew.

Only two of these curios still stood firm. Both were grey, trailing the dirty lace of their porches, swaybacked, pot-bellied and senile. One of them, after its ruined owner had flung himself in front of one of his own trains, had been converted into a warehouse. It now held all the reuttite mantles produced between 1904 and 1929—nearly all the reuttite there was, and representing 25 years of attempts to find some use for it other than gas mantles.

The other house was still, as it had always been, the Smilax house. Phineas Smilax, the first and only president of the Gardnerville, Fernley and New York Railway ("Route of Reuttite"), had invested heavily in the mineral. He had hoped that, as he and Altoona grew richer, the line would actually extend as far east as New York City.

Phineas began building his railroad line in 1885. The work progressed slowly, and this was in part due to certain peculiarities in his hiring policies. Orders existed to fire any man caught beating a horse, drowning a kitten, or tying a can to a dog's tail. He further refused the coolie labour his competitors relied upon, preferring instead bible students, who sang, at his request, hymns while they worked. His favourite hymn was *The Celestial Railroad*. Despite his paying them the then-lavish wage of one dollar an hour, the students were so poorly suited to this work that progress was measured at first in feet per month, then in inches. By 1913, his empire stretched from Altoona to Warm Springs, a fifty-eight-mile vista of sagebrush which he inspected daily in his private car.

This car was the only luxury Phineas permitted himself, for he believed in moderation in all things. The excess of his fortune was always distributed to charities, among which he never scanted the Animal Protection League. Phineas was known to all as a kindly and temperate man—no less to his own children than to strangers. He never chastised his son and daughter by more than a reproving frown, and more was never required.

Perhaps the only fault his neighbours might have found with him was in his choice of servants. Phineas had taken into his employ in the great house in Altoona people from the Nevada Asylum for the Criminally Insane.

"Criminals, pish!" he would exclaim. "They are merely poor unfortunates, languishing for want of a kind word." For over twenty years he had no other servants, and a gentler, more trustworthy set could scarce be found.

One day in 1913 Phineas sat looking out the window of his

private car at the sagebrush, state flower of Nevada. "I feel old, today," he remarked to his secretary, who afterwards remembered it as the first time he had ever heard his master complain. "I feel I'm getting near the end of the line."

The secretary handed him a telegram from his butler, back in Altoona. Phineas Smilax read it and fell from his chair, dead.

The telegram read, "DAUGHTER ENCEINTE REPEAT PREGGERS STOP HAVE BEATEN HER WITH HORSEWHIP AND DRIVEN HER FROM THE TOWN ALTHOUGH I AM FATHER OF THE CHILD STOP PLEASE ADVISE DISPOSITION HER CLOTHING PORTRAIT ETCETERA STOP SIGNED CRAGELL".

The daughter was never found. Cragell, having admitted to raping Lotte and frightening her into silence for several months, was returned to the Asylum. Phineas Jr. took over his father's debts and began his own family, sired on a feeble-minded maid-servant. By his own daughter he had an indeterminate number of children also, and hanged himself in 1930, when the last of the railroad had gone to pay his bootleggers. Three generations of illiterate Smilaxes still lived in the grey house, gardening in its yard. They never spoke of their banished relative, Lotte.

Rusty rails now stretched away from Altoona in three directions. Only the Nevada Southern continued to operate one train a week between Altoona and Las Vegas. Mary Junes Beele had circled on her calendar the day on which that train would leave. Tomorrow was the circled day.

The Beeles had now been here two weeks, and each had made a certain reputation. No one liked Mary. The women did not like the deliberating way she looked over their menfolk. Their menfolk did not like the insolent way she deliberated and rejected them. No one liked the way she treated her husband.

Barthemo, on the other hand, was sought out to about the same degree that Mary was snubbed. He was, after all, the finest gossip the town had ever seen, having already aired one new scandal and dug up a dozen old ones in his first week on the job. As a result of the very first issue of the *Altoona Truth*, two families were not speaking, and there was talk of a divorce, a spite fence, a duel. He reported *everything*, with scrupulous objectivity and in delicious detail. It was said that one day Beele would describe his own cuckolding fairly.

Filled with sweet loathing for her husband, Mary entered the press room, where he was reading a proof.

"Your coperation is appreciated," he read, then paused to add an "o". He did not greet his wife or acknowledge her existence in any way. "... how long will these goings-on continue?" he read, then amended it to "... how long will these goings-on go on?"

"Yaddadda yaddadda go on?" she mocked.

He continued reading.

"No one ever comes to this damned town," she said.

"Nothing ever happens in this damned town," she added.

"The only time we see a fresh face in this damned town," she concluded, "is when someone strays off the road to Vegas."

"What about that hitchhiker? He isn't on the way to Las Vegas, but to the US Navy Ammunition Depot."

"Oh, the sailor. He doesn't count. I'm bored with him already," she said, wrinkling her nose. "Can I use the car tonight, by the way?"

Her husband nodded, not looking up from his proof. "Find out if you can," he said, "why he has those tattoos of Dumbo and Bambi on his arms. There might be a feature story in that—human interest, you know, something for the puzzle page."

That night, while Barthemo Beele was inserting into his paper a late news item about the adultery of an editor's wife, Mary and the sailor were discovering, in the back seat of the Ford, that they were very drunk. The Ford was parked at the edge of town, near the entrance of the Lost Albanian Mine.

"I hear something," mumbled the sailor. "It ain't your old man, is it?"

"Him? Don't worry," Mary said, laying a hand on Bambi. "Listen, he's busy right now, putting the paper to bed. He's some kind of—not freak—neurotic, I guess. All he cares about is putting the damned *paper* to bed. *Altoona Truth*. He wants to bring out a Sunday edition called the *Altoona Altruist*. Faugh!" She took a drink down savagely, then another.

"Shh. Someone out there, baby. Hey, maybe it's the Lost Albanian himself, eh? Ha ha." He poured himself a paper cup of gin and swallowed it. As long as they were this drunk, there seemed no point in stopping.

"Don't even say that joking!" she gasped. "They say if you see the Lost Albanian, the world is coming to an end. Jeesus, that would be a story for Barty, now, wouldn't it? Let's change the subject. Are you gonna take me away on the train tomorrow or not?"

"Sure I am."

A low, blocky shape appeared, ghostly grey, at the dark

entrance to the mine shaft. It scuttled across the moonlit stretch of ground towards them.

"Snakes!" screamed the sailor. "I've gone snakey!"

"You can drink all you want," murmured Mary sleepily. She had not seen the shape. "As long as you take me away from the *Altoona Tooth* ... I mean the ..." She dozed, resting her dirty knot of hair upon Dumbo. The sailor did not notice. He peered fearfully out in the dark, looking for more hallucinations. So this was the DT's! Only a few days before, he had finished his tour of duty at Wompler Research, where all hell had broken loose—little grey boxes. It must be that they were stuck in his unconscious somehow, and the DT's released them, he theorized. Something clanked under the car, but he refused to hear it. He closed his eyes and sipped gin, until, a certain percentage of his blood becoming alcohol, he slept.

At 11:00 the next morning Barthemo Beele and the town marshal woke them up.

"Hey, where's the car?" groaned the sailor.

"We've been robbed!" Mary exclaimed.

Barthemo busied himself taking pictures of the couple from various angles, while the marshal questioned them about the robbery. The four of them compiled a list of the stolen articles:

1 bracelet, ankle, lady's
1 clasp, metal, purse
1 zipper, metal, dress
1 lipstick
1 compact
2 silver dollars and an unknown amount of change, several hairpins
2 cigarette lighters
1 aluminium comb
various keys
2 silver fillings from Mary's teeth
1 gold tooth from sailor
1 automobile, Ford.

"I'll go phone this into the highway patrol, just as soon as the lines are working again," said the marshal. "You know it's a funny thing. Just about every car in town has been stolen. Bicycles, too, and I don't know what-all. And wouldn't you know it, my highway patrol radio transmitter got misplaced too." He wandered off, in the direction of the Town Talk Bar.

"Very interesting," the editor mused. He, too, had been hearing strange rumours and complaints all morning. Now, as he sat down in the grass beside Mary and the sailor, his mind began spinning out headlines for an extra edition:

NO WHEELS? ANTI-CLIMAX

"The telephone lines are down," he murmured. "So are the power lines. Odd."

"I'm leaving you, Barty," Mary said.

"And at least a dozen cars stolen—old cars, too."

"I'm going on the noon train with Lovey," she said firmly. The sailor looked abashed.

"You might think that someone wanted to cut Altoona off from the outside world," Beele said.

"To Las Vegas. I'm not coming back."

"I can assume either that *they* don't want us to know what is going on outside, or—and what is more likely—*they* want to keep those outside from knowing what is going on here. Very odd."

"Monster! Monster!" she screamed, inches from his vacant eyes.

"Now there's an idea," he said abstractedly. "Monsters from outer space have kidnapped us, and we don't know it yet."

He wondered if the Air Force's nearby radar shack knew of the strange phenomenon ... or if they had been affected by it. Whole new panoramas of headlines opened before his inner vision, miles of exclusive copy.

NO RADAR ON?

———

AF WIRELESS

———

We will toast neither our bread nor our power company this a.m. The lines are down. The lines that supply us with power, heat, light, communication, our umbilical cords to the outside world all down. Moreover we are without transportation. There is not a vehicle left in town: not a car, not a bicycle, not so much as a roller skate. Yet even more frightening is the prospect of impairment of our national defence network. How soon are our complacent authorities going to come too, and realize ...

43

Mary and the sailor did not further disturb his reverie. Rising, they dusted themselves off and strolled away in the direction of the station. Barthemo wondered if a sarcastic public notice would be more appropriate.

Due to circumstances beyond, it seems, the control of the city fathers, there will be a slight interruption termination in a few of our public utilities ...

It registered on him then that Mary was gone. *To the station.* But if whoever was cutting off Altoona from the outside world were as thorough as *they* seemed, it was a sure bet *they* would not miss the train. He would take his camera. He would take pictures of *them* actually stealing a train, 60-second pictures, with his new camera.

By one minute to twelve he was hidden under the station platform, his camera beside him. When he had stopped at the office to pick it up, a dozen people had tried to waylay and buttonhole him. There were conflicting stories about the water and gas being cut off, about walking tool boxes—and one intriguing item about poltergeists at the old Ruyteck house, the warehouse for gas mantles.

WHO HAUNTS WAREHOUSE?

Neighbours rattled by ghostly knocks

He could not get over the feeling that he was not alone in the darkness.

The train from Las Vegas, no special, came puffing in a leisurely ten minutes late, took on mail, took on water, took on two passengers, a woman and a sailor, and puffed off again in the direction it had come. Aside from the goggled engineer's waving at the woman passenger as she boarded, nothing seemed odd.

Suddenly there was a crunching sound close at hand. The editor turned to see a large blocky shape beside him, digesting his camera. It seemed to do so with difficulty, as though it were full already, yet it remained in place, while its crab-claw hands picked up every crumb. So this was it!

"Eureka!" he cried, and, as was his habit, unnecessarily translated, "I have found it!" Leaping up joyfully, he brought his head into painful and concussive contact with the bottom of the platform. *What else do metal boxes eat?* he wondered as consciousness fled. *What would I eat, if I were a metal box? Surely not an editor . . . ?*

He awoke some time that afternoon to find the thing no longer beside him. His tongue noted fillings missing, and his belt no longer functioned. No buckle. These were reassurances that he had not been dreaming. *Zap!* Even the metal spring from his note-pad was gone; even the lead from his pencil. He could see the banner now:

GNAWING GNOME PUTS BITE ON TEETH, BELTS BUCKLE

———

Foxy box has goat-like appetite

With maybe a cut of the thing munching a tin can. Barthemo felt he had it made.

Rumours came to meet him as he passed along Park Avenue, and more than rumours. Flying saucers, thousands of fire-breath-ing monsters were solemnly attested to by sober citizens. *Great,* he thought. *Next it'll be a telepath as big as a house.* He gnashed his unfilled teeth on their silly rumours. Barthemo Beele con-sidered himself a lover of truth, stranger to fiction.

Why, it's as though it read my mind! he thought, staring at the Ruyteck house. The poltergeist no longer haunted the building—it had *become* the building. Seemingly the crumbling grey castle had come to life; it tipped and swayed in a clumsy sort of dance. His mind refused to function—except to curse the loss of his camera. Here was a million-dollar picture, and it could only happen in the West, where monsters were monsters.

The worn edifice shivered and rattled obscenely—he thought of the rotting corpse of a dowager doing the twist—and stretched itself upwards, rising, as it were, on tiptoe. Its towers stopped slumping and actually towered, as nails screamed from boards, mould-softened timbers flaked apart, and a century of dust boiled from every crack.

The old house gave a final shudder, shaking off ornaments and pieces of window as if they were drops of water, swayed, tipped up crazily on one corner and—

Disappeared. Came to pieces so suddenly and completely that it was like a vanishing trick. Turned in an instant from a solid build-ing to a pile of flat lumber. A bouncing cluster of bright metal boxes exploded from the remains and skipped about aimlessly, as though getting their bearings. They broke apart and bounced off in different directions, then, but all with seeming purpose. The editor noted one peculiarity about this set of monsters—their surfaces seemed to be made of gas mantles, stuck together in some way.

MARTIAN MONSTERS THE MCCOY

———

Plunder house, don gas mantles

He followed one of the trundling boxes up Park Avenue to the corner of Broadway, where it paused at a fire hydrant.

DOGS WILL BE ALIENS

But the box was *surrounding* the hydrant. It split apart, then closed over it. A moment later there came a small geyser from the assembly. He saw a sort of crude water-wheel, fashioned like a child's pinwheel, spinning in the middle of the jet. A small box detached itself from the assembly and dashed away. Part of its surface, he noted, was of red-painted cast iron.

INVADER WEDS FIREPLUG

———

Can this marriage last?

In the distance the water tower, a giant golf ball on a tee, began to wilt. He watched it dent and collapse, as grey shapes swarmed over it.

AU REVOIR, OUR RESERVOIR

He thought of simply filling up the headline with question marks, but there were not enough in the type case to do so. There were not even enough to take care of all the questions he wanted to put to his readership.

He turned and headed for the office. It was only by chance that he peered in the door of Smilax's Hardware—after all, like all the other buildings on the block, its windows were smashed—but what he saw made him halt.

What he did not see, rather. The store was utterly empty, looted clean. He found the owner, Milo Smilax, lying on the floor at the back, weeping. The metal frames from the bottom halves of his glasses were missing, naturally. He babbled of washing machines. Never a coherent man at best, Milo was now gubbling:

"I'm a dead man, they ruint me! The washing goddamned machines boxes washing machines ruint me eating guns. Help me mama don't tell boxes tell fare thee wellington remington washington ne'er-do-well. They eat the coal scuttling like grabs up anything handy saws gone screws gone knives gone fishing rods the..."

Dr. Trivian would have said the shelves were unfulfilled. In fact, about all that remained were the seed catalogues, the price tags, and a worn, scuffed cardboard sign. Milo stared at the sign as he babbled on. It said, "LOOKING FOR TOOLS?" The pupils of LOOK's eyes were looking at the blank eyes of TOOLS. "SEE OUR SAWS".

"It's the end! Ruint! Nails, saws, chains, everything gone with the w—"

"The end? It is, is it? Is that any way to talk, Milo? I'll admit it looks bad right now, but we haven't got the big picture, have we? I mean, we have to *fight* this thing—or these things—not just lay around crying. We have got to—"

But Milo was not listening; he lay back and resumed crying. "Nails, screws, bolts, saws, keys, hammers, tongs, axes, files, rifles, knives, hooks, shotguns, pistols, axes, guns, knives, bombs, daggers, death..."

"There now," said Beele, edging out the door. "Hang on. I'm sure help is on the way."

The problem, he reflected, was an interesting one. No one knew what to call the invader(s). He would be able to make up a name for them, perhaps add a word to the language. Say, *Uncrobs* (Unidentified Creeping or Crawling Objects).

He filed it away along with the news story about Milo.

HARDWHERE STORE

———

Greedy gadget bites nails, chisels

Before him a little girl sat on the sidewalk, weeping. A naughty dog, she told him, had bit her where she sat down. Moreover she had lost her baby—her 7-transistor radio-doll, that is—to a great big giant. Beele told her not to cry, and that he was sure help was on the way.

He hurried on towards the office. This would be the biggest news story ever, anywhere.

THE BOXES THAT ATE ALTOONA

———

Even the rivets of a child's blue jeans!

A sort of typewriter passed him. It had been broken and distorted, but he could still see the name L. C. Smith on the back plate. Beele swore and broke into a run. A case of type, now became something else, waddled out of his office, brushing him aside at the door, and made its majestic way down the street.

As he entered, Beele seemed to hear the hand-press calling for help. He flung open the door of the press room and rushed in, but too late! The press was already taking on a familiar boxy shape. As he neared it, it gave a final clank, lurched to the window, and fell through into the street. A burglar alarm went off, but was strangled at once.

PAPER RAPED!

The office was stripped clean. How ironic it was, he thought. Unwittingly the machine invaders had destroyed the only means to their justly-deserved fame. Or had they? He rushed out again.

It was after dark by the time he reached a phone booth on the highway that worked. After breaking it open for a dime, he tried to call the wire services. Each time he would get connected, and say, "I'm from Altoo—", the connection would break and his dime rattle back down. He was beginning to wonder whether he hadn't ruined the mechanism somehow, when a highway patrol car stopped. The men in it were not highway patrolmen.

They forced open the door of the phone booth and dragged him forth.

"Sorry to be rough with you, sir," said one, tipping his snap-brim hat. "But our nation's security is at stake. You're Beele, of Altoona? The editor?"

"Yes, but—"

"We've got express orders to keep this particular story quiet, Beele. I'm afraid we'll have to either take you into custody or—"

"Go ahead, kill me!" he said. He, Barthemo Beele, hard-hitting young editor, was weeping. "I have nothing to live for, now. I've

48

lost my press, type fount, wife, typewriter, everything! Go ahead, paid assassins, hirelings of the do-nothing bureaucracy! Kill me! You've already killed the only thing that meant anything to me—my story!"

"I was going to say, we'll either have to take you into custody or swear you in as an agent. We often do that with newsmen, then send them off on foreign assignments. Of course we'll have to investigate your background thoroughly—that'll take an hour or so. What do you say? Would you like to go to Morocco?"

An agent of the CIA! Beele could see it in his mind's eye: palm trees, intrigue, a chance to clean up corruption at the very source!

"I'll take it," he said, smiling through his tears.

CHAPTER VII

THE GULLS OF MARRAKECH

"They four had one likeness, as if a wheel had been in the midst of a wheel."

Ezekiel 10:10

HAROUN AL RASCHID was being difficult, pretending not to understand what Suggs was asking him to sell.

"This puts me in an embarrassing position," he said, sighing *kif* smoke behind his bejewelled hand. "You see, M'sieur Suggs, I do not officially even know of the French mission in this city. How can I give you the information you seek? If you used it, my reputation with the French might be—as you say—battered? I might lose friends, influence—and for what?"

"You must help us," Suggs said grimly. "Give us the name of their man, at least. I know you know it; Haroun knows everything that goes on in Marrakech."

Al Raschid leaned back slightly, his fat mouth rounding in a moue of disavowel. "You flatter me, M'sieur." The tight linen of his suit prevented him from sprawling on the low couch, as he so obviously wished to do; it was with great effort that he moved in any direction, even to reach for his mint tea. "I tell you, it is in my mind to help you, M'sieur Suggs, as a friend helps a friend. But—I do not know. The risk is great."

"You must know *something* of use." The CIA man tried to hold his breath whenever a whiff of *kif* smoke came near, but now he leaned across the low brass table and spoke in an earnest whisper. "Just give us the man's name, that's all. It is for the good of Morocco as well as that of the United S—Nations. The whole world will benefit."

"Ah, but that is what the Russian gentleman says. Which of you is telling the truth?" With a cunning gleam in his eye, Haroun added, "What is a simple man to believe? I am not well-educated. I am only a poor merchant, as you see."

The sweep of his glittering hand indicated the parquet floor, rich carpets, mosaic walls; it took in the stained glass lancets and the delicate, jewel-like chandeliers. The room was a chaos of textures: brass, wood, leather, silk, wool, silver, velvet. Through a marble doorway Suggs could see the cool garden where a white peacock stalked to and fro beneath the lemon trees.

"As you see, I have not the air conditioning. I have not the television set. I have none of the luxuries so commonplace in your land, no, not even the electric toothbrush."

Hiking up his jelaba, Suggs brought out a slim billfold. "We are prepared to pay, of course," he said. "Anything reasonable."

"Ah!" Haroun's tiny nostrils exhaled twin jets of aromatic smoke. "Then I must overcome the scruple of my conscience. Here is the right half of a picture of the man you seek. His name is Brioche, Marcel Brioche. He is a pilot of planes for the French Air Force—and who knows what else, eh?"

"No one is exactly what he seems," Suggs said pleasantly. As his left hand reached out to take the half-picture his right, still inside his jelaba, fired his silenced gun. Haroun Al Raschid did not move, but only grunted slightly as the front of his silk shirt grew purple with blood.

Suggs did not wait to see the inevitable look of surprise on his victim's face—after nine years in the CIA, one grew weary of such looks—but tucked the photo in his billfold and hurried out into the sun-drenched street. He drew up his hood as he ran. The motion set scalding pangs of diarrhoea growling in his guts.

A crowd of ragged boys besieged him almost at once, and followed him to his hotel, chanting:

"M'soo, M'soo! You want gull, nice gull? You want nice boy? *Kif*, smoke? Mister! 'Allo! You like picture? You like see dancing gull? You like camel whip? Me very strong, M'soo! You want shoes shine? Me guide, M'soo. Me guide. You want nice gull?"

His disguise had not been as effective as he had hoped.

In the lobby, Suggs bought a postcard depicting snake charmers in the market, Dar El Fna, and a stamp. "Dear Madge," he wrote. "Still having wonderful time, though I miss you and Susie. Love, Bubby." He mailed it at the desk.

Scotty, his partner, sat in the only comfortable chair in their room, reading an Arabic newspaper. "Did you get it?" he asked, without glancing up. Suggs nodded as he locked the door. "Good man. Haroun give you any trouble?"

"A little. I had to kill him."

"That's tough. We could have used him. What happened?"

"Tell you as soon as I get the report made out, Scotty." Divesting himself of the jelaba and loosening his tie, Suggs sat down at the portable and rolled in a triplicate form.

"Item: one bullet, .375 calibre," he typed. "Date used; 1 June, 196–." He went on, typing slowly, taking a certain pride in his neat spacing. When he had finished, he brought out the half-photo and showed it to Scotty.

"He was going to sell *them* the other half," Suggs explained.

The other looked surprised. "Them? I thought Vovov was working alone on this."

"Not any more. This is too big for just Vovov. They know as well as we do what's going on here—that this Brioche is an astronaut—that France means to put him on the moon. They've brought in their top man, Vetch. Maybe to check on his subordinate, or maybe to finger this Brioche."

"How do you know Vetch is in town?"

Suggs wagged a finger playfully. "Oh, I have my spies, I have my spies," he said. "But what worries me is, have they *already* got the other half of this? Do they know what Marcel Brioche looks like?"

"Are you sure he's the man?"

Suggs nodded. "We've got to contact him before they offer him —the moon."

Neither man smiled. They lapsed into a thoughtful silence, each trying to unravel the mystery surrounding the half-picture.

—Why had Haroun offered him only half a picture? Suggs wondered. It didn't make sense, if he had intended to sell the other half to the Russians. Perhaps he only had meant to hold it back for more money. Haroun was too smart to try selling to both sides.

But there were other things that did not make sense. What of the crowd of urchins—they had recognized him through his disguise as an American! Could they have stolen the other half of the picture? What kind of pictures had *they* been trying to sell him? He recalled their grimy, skinny hands clutching at him—could they have picked his pocket? Perhaps, on the other hand, they had been trying to warn him of something—of the location of the rocket, for example. What was it they had said about gulls? "You want gull?" But Marrakech was in the middle of the desert, hundreds of miles from any gulls! It was a code, then, but a code for what, he could not imagine. He was about to ask Scotty, when something, a gleam of scrutinizing eye, arrested him. What was Scotty thinking about?

—Scott watched his partner watching him. Yes, there was guilt in Suggs's face, real guilt and worry. He had killed today, almost for no reason. Then too, he was reticent about his sources of information. How had he found out what the Russkies were up to? What was going through his mind now? Scott was glad he had taken the precaution of tucking his gun down the side of his chair earlier.

—If the urchins had seen through his disguise, Suggs reasoned, only one person could have tipped them off—the only person who knew about his visit this afternoon—Scotty! His partner in the CIA for nine fantastic years!

Suddenly, Suggs knew fear. Was Scotty hiding a gun behind that Arab paper? Well, there was always the typewriter. Its carriage could fire a single shotgun shell—Scotty had probably forgotten that.

It seemed incredible that Suggs' partner could have sold out, but he must have done so. To whom? Suggs wondered. Not to the Russians, or he'd have known about Vetch. Was he, then, working for Morocco? For France? Or was he playing some even deeper game?

—What kind of game was Suggs playing? Scott wondered. Had he killed Haroun because the merchant knew too much? Had Haroun called him outright a double agent? There was no doubt Suggs was a wheel within a wheel, but for whom? He wondered how he could have let Suggs fool him for so long. Why, everything about him gave it away—the half-picture, the over-casual way he seemed to be looking at the ashtray, while his other hand was out of sight, going for a gun.

—There were no ashes, Suggs noted, but there had been ashes yesterday. Someone had cleaned this ashtray. Why? He saw the over-casual way Scotty was yawning. Was he getting ready to make his play?

—Was Suggs making his play?

—Yes, *now!*

—*Now!* Fire through the newspaper!

—*Now!* Suggs stabbed the question mark button on the typewriter.

Fire and steel exploded. Scotty slumped forward, dead.

"I'm really sorry, Scotty," Sugg murmured, standing over the corpse. "I wish you could get a hero's funeral, at least. But I gotta protect myself, old shoe. The noise of that shotgun blast will bring the police. I've got to make sure the hotel will pay them off and cover up your death."

He opened an emergency kit and dug out a black lace brassiere and a lipstick. He fastened the brassiere about the cadaver's torn chest and drew red upon the discoloured lips. Then he looked hard at the half-photo, memorized the address on the back, tore it in bits and swallowed them.

Heavy footsteps sounded on the stairs as he left by the balcony. Suggs took a last look at the body.

"Don't worry, Scotty," he said earnestly. "I'll get the bastards for making me do this. So help me."

CHAPTER VIII

THE END OF THE WORLD

*"What are little girls made of? Contain dextrose, maltose,
monosodium glutamate, artificial flavouring and colour-
ing; sodium propionate added to retard spoilage."*

Old Saying

THOUGH THE TELEVISION newscaster seemed hysterical,
Susie Suggs was not agitated in the least. She was not really
watching the screen of her portable TV; it served only as a flat
weight on her tummy, while she did her deep breathing exercises
according to *Lady Fair* magazine. The exercises made her sleepy,
and the voice of the little figure seemed to dwindle to a mosquito
hum. It was almost as if he were a little man growing right out of
her tummy; but this idea was so vaguely disquieting that it
brought her fully awake. Forgetting to count her breaths, Susie
began actually watching.

"Is it a Russian sneak attack? Is it one of our own secret weapons gone somehow horribly wrong? Or is it something we are
even less prepared to face—an invasion of beings not of this
planet? We'll have the whole story in just a moment, after this
message from the Vortex Corporation."

The screen went white, then displayed a large white missile
sitting in a mesh of black iron railings. Fire swelled from under
it as, trembling, the giant cylinder rose into darkness.

"This is . . . the Moloch!" intoned a solemn announcer. "America's newest power punch! Just look at this baby go!" The missile
rose, tilted, and headed off into the night. "Now watch the Moloch
destroy this mock-up of an enemy village!" Something white
flashed downward into a grass village, and both exploded together
—*"Wow!"* said the announcer—in one instant of blinding glare.

The scene changed to a complicated laboratory, where a group
of men in white coats listened to earphones and watched, on a
dozen little TV screens, the destruction re-enacted.

"These capable, experienced men designed Moloch. They are
the members of Vortex Missile Group, just one of Vortex's 'Keep
America Tough' programmes. Every man here is a genius,
dedicated and committed to our ever-expanding missile pro-

gramme. They have solved the launch and guidance problems of the Moloch—and of *seventeen other* military missiles. Yes, at Vortex, retaliation is a way of life.

"Vortex is many things to many people. Here we see a steel mill run by computers from Vortex Instrument Group. And here", he said, and Susie took more interest in the next scene, for it was an operating room, "here is Dr. Toto Smilax performing open heart surgery—using a scalpel made by Vortex Cutlery Group.

"*Vortex!*" exclaimed the announcer in conclusion. "First in war and first in peace—and first in the hearts of its countrymen."

The newscaster returned. "Altoona, Nevada," he said. "Until today, just another ordinary American city in the West. Now—who knows? Life *may* be going on as usual in Altoona—*as far as we know*. But since early this morning there has been a news blackout imposed by the joint efforts of the FBI, the CIA and the National Security Agency. We have been unable to contact anyone within the city.

"What has happened? Frankly, we don't know. It could be, as some hint, a Russian invasion, or even an invasion from outer space. Calmer sources believe it to be a test of some sort, and at least one reliable source indicated that it might be a secret weapon gone wrong. *We just don't know*." Every time he used this phrase, the newscaster's face seemed a little more crumpled, a little closer to tears. For another fifteen minutes he told Susie of all the things we don't know. Then the announcer with the soothing voice (that sent nice warm ripples over Susie's tummy) returned to demonstrate the two-stage Hermes-Aphrodite missile. Advertising was so silly, Susie thought, resuming her breathing exercises.

By her *Lifetime* watch, she noted how late it was getting. She was going to have to hustle to be ready for her date with Ron. And she had meant to study for her Organic Chem test Monday morning. Here it was Saturday night and she hadn't opened the book!

Quickly Susie showered with *Nice*, the 24-hour soap that gets at odours other soaps just seem to miss, and rolled on plenty of SHUR, to be sure about those offensive odours. After dusting all over with Lady Clinge talc, she slipped on her *Modaform* 6-way-stretch panty girdle that b-r-e-a-t-h-e-s, her Deepline *Modaform* Sport-support bra, and began applying *Classique* Parfum, the scent that makes every woman an empress, every man a slave.

Drawing on her black sweater and black skirt, Susie seated

herself at the vanity table to do her face. After covering her golden freckles with *Blanc* foundation, she powdered with Rubella Gorne's *Klown* powder. To her Greekly perfect mouth, she applied a white lipstick called *Eraser*.

For her eyes, Susie selected her usual assortment of Nora Hart shades, chiefly oyster and sylph-green, but blending in touches of burgundy and bronze. Then, after brushing her hair and applying a liberal amount of *Airnet,* there remained only jewellery.

On a velvet bar in Susie's vanity kit were pinned Bob's △KE pin, Len's Young Republican pin, and Jim's Vietnam button. Her fingers passed over these, nor paused at the Pepsi *Come Alive!,* the *Go Gophers!,* or the *Win With Dewey* buttons, went on to the end of the bar and selected the peace mandala Ron had given her. As she pinned it on, her mother came to the door.

"That awful creature Ron is here," she stage-whispered. "Oh, I'm sorry I don't like him, dear, but he's so—so shifty. And he always wears old clothes. And now—now he's even growing a *beard!* Ugh!"

Fighting down her own repulsion at the idea, Susie said, "But mother, he's one of the richest boys in the city of Santa Filomena. Surely you want me to have a good future?"

"I don't know. I just don't know." Madge's tanned face deepened its seams with worry. "I married your father because he had a good future with the insurance company. Now look at me."

Susie looked at her mother and saw an attractive middle-aged woman right from the pages of *Lady Fair,* to which Madge subscribed: dark hair, streaked with silver, a slim, girlish figure, and the only clue to her years being the lines in her face. Susie fervently wished that she herself, at thirty-five, would look as good.

Madge went on, "I guess I shouldn't try to tell you how to run your life, after I've made such a mess of my own. Every time I think of that bastard—how he's enjoying himself over there with his harem girls—not even a postcard, in over three months! Well, I saw the lawyer today, and I'm suing him for a divorce. If he can live it up, so can I! Sauce for the goose! While the cat's away!"

Madge seemed to have been drinking. She lurched to the mirror and examined her eyes, pulling the loose flesh beneath them this way and that. She scarcely seemed to notice that Susie had drawn on her white felt boots, kissed her goodbye and said, "That's the spirit, Mommy! Kick him in the—the seater! 'Bye."

Near the campus of the University of California, at Santa Filomena, one street featured four well-patronized coffee houses, but none so popular as The Blue Tit. To avoid difficulties with university officials the owner of the coffee house, Kevin Mackintosh, had painted a bluebird on the café's sign. As on all weekend nights, a crowd had crammed itself into The Blue Tit to listen to folk music and poetry, but tonight it was a sullen, heavy-spirited crowd. Many of them had arrived, as had Susie and Ron, on motorcycles in the drizzle, and the room was filled with steam and the sour smell of wet wool.

On a raised dais at the rear of the narrow room, a poet was reading aloud from a sheet of paper held close to his face. As he turned to catch the light, Susie recognized Kevin Mackintosh.

"*Timepoem* number fourteen," he read.

> "*Johnson in Omaha: loud ticks from the inner clock.*
> *There always has to be a victim*
> *In cool and secret stride*
> *No motives other than patriotism*
> > *and pure disgust.*
> *Back to business, without boots.*
> *Look here for an explosive spirit.*"

"Golly!" Susie exclaimed. "Explosives reminds me, I ought to be studying for that Organic Chem test Monday."

"Ssh," said Ron. "There isn't going to be any day after tomorrow."

"I don't know the Geneva naming system or anything."

Ron smiled. Kevin Mackintosh looked at her, incredulous. "The Geneva naming system is done," he said. "So is the Geneva convention. So is Geneva."

"It's the end of the world," Ron explained.

"That's right," said someone else. "The crack of doom has been sounded."

"What do you mean?" asked Susie, smiling a little. "I don't get it."

"It's the end of the whole works, baby," Ron said. "Like they tell us on the radio. Didn't you hear the news?"

"This is our end-of-the-world party," announced Kevin Mackintosh, "Bring your own."

Someone snickered, but the poet was not smiling.

"Will someone please tell me what this is all about?" Susie asked. She thought and thought, but was unable to recall just what she had seen on the six o'clock news.

"That thing in Altoona, Nevada," Ron explained, "is either a Russian missile, Something Horrible from outer space, or one of our own screaming nightmares. If it is a Russian missile, we retaliate. Then they retaliate. Et cetera, the end.

"If it is a thing from outer space, why does the government keep it so quiet? Because it is something pretty horrible, like a thing that digested the whole town, or atomic monsters, shooting X-rays all over. Something we can't stop, that'll take over.

"If it is some weapon of our own out of control, what would it be? Some bomb? Not likely, or other countries would be raising hell. More likely a nasty disease—say universal contagious cancer."

Everyone in the room had grown silent. It was as if they huddled together in the gloom actually waiting for a quick blinding light to illumine and transfigure them for one final instant. The most important actions and words were pointless; the most trivial were full of meaning, elevated almost to sacraments.

Tears came to Susie's eyes. It all seemed so unfair. She was seventeen years old and still a virgin, and now it was too late. She wanted more than anything to give up pointless, silly virtue now, near the end of All, but it was somehow too small a sacrifice (then, too, there was always the outside chance that the world would *not* end—and then how in the world would she explain things to Madge?). Susie hated the old End-of-the-world suddenly and furiously. She wanted to just scratch its eyes out!

"Why—why I think we ought to go out and protest!" she declared, standing up. The others looked at her, not catching her meaning. "They have no right to do this to us! They have no right to take away the world like this, the selfish pigs!"

There was a sudden high-pitched explosive laugh from one youth. "What do you think we ought to do about it?" he mocked. "Write our congressmen?"

"No," she said seriously. "But I don't think we'll solve anything by just sitting around here moping, for Pete's sake! We ought to go out and—and protest! We ought to march on this Alt—this wherever it is and tell them what we think of them, in no uncertain terms!" She stamped her little boot. "Or are we going to let them take *everything* away?"

The room was in an uproar. Some people were egging her on, while others were thinking over her words. Susie's scorn was magnificent. In vain did someone try to point out that protest against the inevitable is useless.

"Well of course it's useless," she snapped. "I'm not as dumb as all that! But it certainly isn't any use just sitting around here just—steaming, is it?"

"I think she has something," said Ron, grinning. "Why the hell not go down there and protest? It's only ten hours' drive."

"Protest what?" asked Kevin. "The end of the world?"

"Sure, why not?" Ron said. "Like in *Attack of the Fungamen*, everyone protested the dangerous experiments, right? Like in *Goz*, they demonstrate against the army's impotence, remember? And in *The Day the Earth Caught Cold*—"

"All right, all right, but what are we protesting?" Kevin asked. "If I may be so stupid."

"How about the sealing off of an American city by the CIA, and the violations of freedom of speech involved? Come on, we'll make some signs, and we'll get some people who have cars in on this."

Kevin gave in. "We'll let your girl run the show," he suggested. "It was her idea. But I never thought I'd spend my last hours making signs."

"Or getting arrested," Ron added. "The friends won't like this at all."

"If I see any fuzz," said the poet, "I'm going to suddenly have a business deal in Tangier. I'll only go so far for a joke."

It may have been a joke to him and to most of those present (behaving in conscious or unconscious parody of old movies— "Gee gang," someone said, "how are we going to raise money for uniforms for the team?" "I have it! We'll put on an end of the world!"), but to Susie, it meant becoming for a moment a kind of Joan of Arc. As they left the coffee house, she was at the fore, her white boots lifting high, higher, leading the parade.

Certainly Madge never worried less about the vincibility of her daughter's innocence than now, having just heard her insist on the word "seater", and seeing her blush as she pronounced it. How innocent Susie was, and how wise she herself had been at that age.

Madge was now only dimly aware of the dying roar of Ron's Harley, only vaguely cognizant of her own hand, caressing the buttons on the velvet bar in Susie's vanity kit. Madge was seeing herself of eighteen years ago, going out to the Webster Beach Club with a handsome young insurance salesman.

How like the youthful Suggs was one of Susie's friends, Jim Porteus, she thought. Odd that Susie never noticed it in him. He was such a nice boy—so earnest, in his glasses with their customary rims of solemn black, so energetic, so eager to set the world on fire. Madge fingered the yellow pin he'd given Susie: "NO RETREAT—BEAT THE VIET CONG."

Jim was already worth money in his own right, besides being the son of a prominent gynaecologist, and leader of the California chapter of *Young Americans to Conserve Free Enterprise.*

When he was serious, he was serious indeed. Madge recalled every detail of the first conversation she'd had with him:

"Are you planning on studying medicine yourself, Mr. Porteus?"

"No I'm not, Mrs. Suggs." He removed the glasses, startling her with the hard planes of his face. "No, I'm afraid the medical profession is a dead letter, these days. Despite all our efforts to prevent it, socialized medicine is on the way—and with it, *starvation for doctors.*

"No, I've been keeping an ear to the ground while I pursue a course of business administration. Market analysis seems very promising—very promising, I can assure you. Qualified analysts are in short supply. It's an uncrowded field, where an energetic, get-up-early young man can soon make his pile. Or I may opt for corporation law—chiefly protecting infant industries from the predations of the federal eagle—or some related field. I suppose the truth lies somewhere between the two. I may become an humble junior executive, an unknown but vital cog in middle management—a job where the rewards are not mere fiscal aggrandizement, but full commitment to the judicious use of power. I distribute work and rewards—and punishments—to my subordinates, while receiving my own just portion from the higher-ups; a vital link in the Great Chain of Command!"

In many ways, she reflected, thinking back on that conversation, Jim seemed older than her husband.

Madge was shocked to note the time. In the next five minutes she was a flurry of activity, bathing, perfuming, arranging her hair, and enveloping her body in diaphanous pyjamas of mysterious misty grey barely before the bell rang. She hurriedly pinned on the yellow button and ran to greet Jim.

"Wow!" he said. "Is it dark in here! Let's get a little light on the subject."

"Wow!" he repeated, looking her over in the light. "You look great, Madge." He took off his Tyrolean hat and kissed her.

As he undressed, neatly and efficiently, Jim talked of the coming elections for student government, in which his Student Ultra-Conservatives, newly-formed, hoped to win a few seats.

"We're young and dynamic, though inexperienced," he said, folding his socks carefully and hanging them over the back of a chair. "The older parties will just have to move over and make room for us."

Madge moved over and made room for him in the bed.

Woody sat in the dispatcher's office the same night, staring unseeingly at the Lost Property form before him. For hours, he had found himself unable to even begin his strange report—though he saw every detail of it clearly, again and again.

By the time he had brought his little train to a halt that afternoon, the rest of the crew had been on the ground, running for the dispatcher's office where the beer was kept. The Altoona-Las Vegas run always stopped here at Double Flats for beer, especially on hot days. Officially, of course, they stopped to pick up train orders.

"Where's the beer?" asked Fats, the brakeman cheerily.

"I ain't your slavey!" screamed the dispatcher, who never spoke in any other tone. "You know where we keep it! You guys don't know what work is. You don't know how lucky you got it, being out there in the fresh air. I wish I was back on the road, I wish to God I was." He spat into a dim, littered corner, where there might have been a spittoon. Woody and the crew opened beer cans and settled in various creaky chairs about the dark brown room. They were not anxious to get back into the desert dust and heat, no matter how lucky they had it.

Railroading was new and wonderful to Woody, though he pretended to hate it as much as everyone else seemed to do. He was already picking up railroad jargon, such as the differences between boxes, gons, reefers and flats, but he had much to learn. One thing which continued to surprise him was that he did not have to steer the engine. It seemed almost to guide itself, in some way he could not yet fathom, around even the sharpest curves. The railroad was a wonderful invention, he certainly had to admit.

The Nevada Southern was the only railroad he could find still running steam locomotives. Woody would not run any other kind. He loved the heat, the hiss of steam.

"That's right," he put into conversation. "Anyone is crazy to go railroading." The others nodded.

"I'm gonna get out," said Fats. "I got a brother in the feed grain business, I'm gonna go in with him. Feed grain, that's where the real money is."

"I laud that," said Woody solemnly. "The fratricidal bond." The beer had cooled him off and made him feel clear-headed. Earlier, in Altoona, he had suffered an hallucination, no doubt from the heat. A classic wish-fulfilment dream, it had been—a woman he had once known, in another state, seemed to board his train at Altoona. He had even waved at the hallucination, but, being only an hallucination, it had not waved back.

He finished his beer, drew on his gauntlets, and strode to the door. And stopped.

Mac, the fireman stood on the platform, utterly dazed. Fats and the conductor were hopping and sprinting across the tracks towards the train.

The train was moving. It was moving and accelerating, with the throttle wide open.

But the throttle could not be wide open. There was no one in the cab to open it. There was no one to fire the boiler. For all practical purposes, the cab was empty.

Roaring and chattering, slipping, the engine, the coal tender and the single passenger car moved out. The hallucinatory woman seemed to be still aboard.

Fats puffed to a halt. The conductor made a try for the tail end of the car, missed, and fell. He rolled clear as the last wheels nipped by.

A mirage? Mass hypnosis?

Woody dipped the steel pen in ink and scratched upon the form.

"NAME: Elwood Trivian, Ph.D. TITLE: Engineer. ITEM LOST: One train. DESCRIBE THE CIRCUMSTANCES: Apparently the train was stolen, by a—" he lined out "a" and wrote, "by what seemed to be a small, grey tin tackle box."

CHAPTER IX

COINCIDENCE

*"Men that hazard all
Do it in hope of fair advantages."*

SHAKESPEARE

THE YOUNG MAN at the end of the bar was not wearing Western clothes. Had he worn no clothes at all he could not have appeared more conspicuous, at least in *The El Cantina Bar* in Goodtime, Nevada. The *El,* as regulars called it, catered to the brightly-clad guests of three dude ranches. There were the ovoid, unhappy women of the Merry Widow Rancho (awaiting divorces); the unhappy, ovoid men of the Triple-Tumblebug Ranch (awaiting divorces); and the querulous, dozing old people, of no particular sex, from the Golden Sunset Retirement Ranch (awaiting death). Amid their orchids, turquoises and clarets, all the hues of a painted sunset, Cal's rumpled grey suit and dirty-white lab coat stood out like a bird-dropping.

Hitchhiking towards California, he had made it this far before sun, sand, wind, shimmering pavement and truck smoke had driven him indoors.

"Another one?" asked the bartender, poising his bottle. His name, stitched in violet letters over the pocket of his carnelian shirt, was *Slim.* His unlabelled customer nodded solemnly.

"I will have another. And pour yourself another, too, Slim."

"Why, thank you, Carl. Your health."

"It's *Cal.* Say, Slim, tell me, who are all those old people along the wall?"

Slim explained about "retirement ranches". "They come in now and then for a little fun, with their attendants." He indicated a group of bored-looking young men and women at the middle of the bar, all wearing black ten-gallon hats and shirts of ochre silk. On the back of each shirt was embroidered a setting sun, or rising sun, emitting heavy black rays. The attendants' names were stitched in black over their hearts.

"Another thing. How come everything here seems to be made of wagon wheels and barrels? Tables and chandeliers and ... Where do all the wagon wheels come from?"

Slim moved down the bar, smiling, to wait upon two middle-aged women.

"Oh Slim, you *beast!*" shrilled the thin woman in a black-and-lavender shirt. "We've been waiting for *hours!*"

Her friend, a dumpling in oriflamme orange, called Slim a bad boy, and told him she didn't know whether she wanted a frozen Daquiri or not, from such a bad boy. Wasn't he a bad boy, though? she asked her companion.

On the colour television a parade in Texas appeared: whole troops of cowgirls in sky blue, their white boots moving like pistons in synchronous high-kicking steps. The men from the Triple Tumblebug wet their lips and began to chuckle.

Cal had another drink. Two swarthy strangers came in. The smaller was Cal's height, the larger was a giant. They wore Palm Beach suits with wide shoulders and trim straw hats with narrow brims. Nevertheless, their eyes seemed to be in shadow. Cal would have taken them to be policemen, but they were drinking, and top-shelf whiskey, too. There was something familiar about the larger man....

"Another one, Carl?" Slim poured him another, took the proper amount from the jumbled pile of change in front of Cal, and added another receipt to the neat, squared-up stack. An increase or was it decrease in entropy—or was it enthalpy? Cal tried to remember Dr. Trivian and Appreciation of Thermodynamics, but his thoughts were running into ellipses....

He watched the old people along the wall, dozing over cribbage or Monopoly boards and beer. Now and then one would awaken slightly to say something cross, then drift off without waiting for a reply.

The taller of the two newcomers, who reminded Cal somehow of jock-straps, had turned his back, but the shorter man materialized at Cal's elbow. "Pardon me, sir," he said shyly. "My friend and I have a little bet going. I say you're a doctor, and he says you drive a meat truck. I wonder if you'd mind telling me which of us is correct?"

Cal smiled modestly, if crookedly. "Actually, I'm a biophysicist. So I'd say your guess was closer."

"Very interesting." The stranger reamed one ear with a thick finger. "I suppose you know a lot about mathematics, eh?"

"Bingo!" screamed an old person of indeterminate sex, who sat before a cribbage board.

Reluctantly, Cal admitted that he had a nodding aquaintance with the Calculus.

"I see. Well, thanks for settling our bet." The stranger moved off, before Cal could ask him the name of his tall companion. "Tennessee" came to mind, as did "tennis shoe". Cal settled for the moment on something between Dennis Shoe and Jack Strapp....

He realized he was shouting all this when Slim turned and smiled at him. "Keep it down to a dull roar, now, Carl old buddy."

"Cheat!" someone along the wall squeaked. "Where did that hotel come from, eh? Tell me that!"

"You watch your mouth," came the quavering reply. "I own Boardwalk and Park Place, and by the Living God, you'll pay me my rent!"

"Please," said another, an old woman in a scarlet shirt. "Andy can take his turn over, can't he?"

A glass of beer went over. "Now see what you've made me do! All the Chance cards ruined!"

"I'll show *you* who cheats!" screamed a wispy old man in a tall white sombrero and a shirt of distress-signal pink. Above the green neckerchief, his goitre worked convulsively. "There!" He leapt up and whipped the blanket off his opponent's lap. A number of cards fell out of it. "Hah!" he screamed. "Caught with the goods! So that's what happened to all the railroads, eh?"

The culprit, a parrot-like man in blue and orange, picked up a tiny red block of wood and flung it at him. "Take your hotel and go to Hades!" he wailed. Clawing at the board, he upset it, sweeping off hotels, houses, dice and markers. "*You* cheat, yourself!"

"... take his turn over, now, couldn't he, Edna?"

"Cheat! Hah! Sneak!"

"I'll cheat you, by the Living God!" shrieked the man in the hat. He brought up a cane suddenly and began laying about him. "All of you cheated me. All of you cheated me."

There was a stir at the bar, among the group of attendants. One young man spun about on his stool. Above his pocket Cal could make out the name. "Dr. Michaels". He was across the room in three strides, flipping the cane from the old man's hand.

"Now, Toby. Now, Toby, it's only a game," he said.

The old man rolled his eyes and whinnied, "You're all cheating me!"

The doctor drew his black, pearl-handled revolver, pressed the muzzle to Toby's upper arm, and squeezed the trigger.

The two swarthy strangers reached inside their jackets.

Toby visibly relaxed, and his muttering grew faint. Dr. Michaels withdrew the gun. It was, Cal could see, made of black plastic. One might almost take it for a toy, if not for the inch of glittering needle projecting from the barrel. Retracting this, the doctor holstered his weapon.

"Sorry about the disturbance," he grinned to the crowd at large. The hands of the two strangers came out of their jackets, and they laughed foolishly. Dr. Michaels and another attendant lowered the unconscious old man into a wheelchair. Cal saw that it had wagon wheels.

"What are you supposed to be?" a woman in purple demanded of Cal. "Little country doctor? What's the white coat for?"

"In Japan," he tried to say, "white is for mourning."

"In Jamp," he said distinctly, "wise firm? Awning."

Her empurpled lips took a sip of cocktail. With obvious enjoyment she sneered, "Don't hand me that crap! You ain't no doctor! You're just some monkey from the meat market. Why don't you just get back to your pig's feet?"

Cal shook his head, then looked at his feet, trying to puzzle out her meaning. "Why don't I—?"

"You're a mess!" she screamed, spraying spittle. "A mess! Just like my old man. Boy, he was a real bastard. Used to rub grime deliberatedly into his shirts. Used to come home in his filthy shoes and *walk all over the floors*. Put his filthy ashes into every ashtray in the house. Well I had enough of that rotten bastard, and I had enough of you!"

Her cocktail was cold and frothy with cream. Its impact drove him back a few blind steps. Rebounding from a table, he fell. Angry red faces looked down at him. Four or five voices gabbled at once about that man bothering you ma'am, about drunken young snot ought to be in the army, about impersonating a doctor. Hands dragged Cal to his feet.

"About time you were shoving off, old buddy Carl," chortled Slim, steering him towards the door.

"It's *Cal*," he pleaded. "You wouldn't like it if I called you *Slime*, would you?"

"Is that the way you're gonna be?" Slim rabbit-punched Cal and seized his collar. The other hand twisted in the back of his belt. "I knew you was gonna be trouble when you come in here." The door flew towards them.

"But I only meant—"

Cal shot through the door, bounced on all fours, and rolled to rest against a brick wall.

Moonlight streamed down into the alley. Cal lay there awhile, getting his bearings. He saw a number of garbage cans, a poster announcing a Wheelchair Squaredance at the Golden Sunset Ranch, and his own shoeless foot.

Rising painfully, he limped about till he found the missing shoe. When he had finished being sick into it, he put it on.

It was difficult to walk on two legs, so he progressed on four to the alley entrance. The two strangers in Palm Beach suits were waiting for him. Without a word, they picked him up and dumped him in the back of a car. Though it was too dark to tell, Cal felt sure it was a black Cadillac sedan. The shorter man climbed in beside him, while the other slid behind the wheel. He certainly reminded Cal of someone in his graduation class, now two weeks past. But who? Not Barthemo Beele. Not Mary Junes, either....

"Where we going?" he asked, struggling to sit up. The stranger pushed him back in the seat and drew a gun.

"You're being kidnapped, actually, sir. 'The Professor' has given orders to kidnap a mathematician."

"What professor? I wanta see the squealchair wheredance."

"Put this over your eyes, please." He was handed a band of black cloth.

"Does that gun have needle in it, too?"

The others laughed richly. "That's right," growled the driver. "A needle to put you to sleep with—for a long time. Unless you want to take the big sleep, you better do as we—like we say. In this racket, we play for keeps, odd man out, loser take nothing, see?"

There was something familiar about that voice, Cal thought, but by now the blindfold was in place. They drove off.

Five minutes later, after a complicated series of turns, they stopped and hustled him into a building.

"Well, well, well," boomed a hearty voice. "Company already, eh? I suppose this is our mathematician." Cal imagined a cigar-smoking executive gangster rubbing his hands. "Take off the mask and let's have a look at the face of him."

The blindfold was removed, and Cal found himself facing a buxom, pleasant-faced blonde wearing a ruffled mobcap and flannel nightie. She might have stepped out of a Dutch genre painting, but for the fact that she held, not a candle, but a bottle of scotch and a glass. "Welcome to Castle Rackrent!" she boomed. "Care for a drink?"

His stomach contracted. "I don't—think so. Are you—the Professor?"

"Me? Haha, bless you, no, I'm Daisy, the Professor's fiancée and
former secretary. *This* is the Professor."

She moved to one side, revealing a thin, wispy man sitting on
the sofa. His sparse hair, the colour of pounce, lay in dusty streaks
across his baldness. He seemed to be engrossed in writing
with a quill pen in an old, battered book so huge it hid most of
his body, though Cal could see gaitered legs below it. They did
not reach to the floor.

"How do you do?" Cal said.

"How do you—?" creaked the other. But Daisy moved in front
of him like a curtain once more, and he fell silent.

"His real name is Brian Gallopini," she said, pouring herself
a glass of liquor. "But in the Underworld everyone with a college
education gets called 'Professor', you see."

"Then he isn't one, really?"

She drank off the gill and poured herself another. "Oh yes, he's
a professor, all right. Of eighteenth-century literature. Or was. I
was his secretary. We decided to run away and be gangsters, when
he got his idea—but that's another story. My name is Daisy le
Duc, and if you know what's good for you, you'll resist the temptation to call me 'Daisy Duck'." The mirth went out of her smile for
a moment, then returned full-strength. "I'll finish up these intro-
ductions now, then you can go clean the dirt and blood off your
face so we can have a good look at you.

"These are the Professor's associates in crime, Mr. John
Beaumains, known as Jack the Ripper (for no good reason that
anyone can think of), and 'Harry the Ape', whose real name is—"

"Harry Stropp!" The exclamation burst from Cal, who just
that moment had turned and recognized his kidnapper.

Harry, for it was indeed he, peered in bewilderment at the
blood-and-dirt-encrusted face. "Calvin Potter!" he cried. "What
are *you* doing here?"

"I might ask you the same question. Harry, have you gone in
for a life of crime?"

From behind Daisy came a creaky voice. "It is just such coincidences that prove there is a thing called Destiny, presiding
over our so-called 'chance' universe. I'll make a note of that
in my journal." The goose-quill scratched.

"Don't worry," Harry said in a low, confiding tone, "about taking Mary Junes away from me. Oh, it upset me for a while, I'll

69

admit, but I'm all over that, now. There's plenty of other apples on the tree."

"Well now," Daisy chuckled, "let's not keep Mr.—Potter, is it?—Mr. Potter up all night. We're all getting an early start in the morning, for Las Vegas. So I guess I'd better explain why we kidnapped you.

"The Professor has devised an elaborate and foolproof system for beating the wheel. We are going to—figuratively speaking—take Las Vegas by storm. This system can't fail. By this time next week, we should have the key to the city—literally speaking."

"But where do I come in?"

"Exactly!" piped the Professor. "Where do you come in? It seems my system is perfect in theory—that is, the *whole* of it is perfect—but the calculations involved in placing any one bet are too complex for any of us. That is where you, our Mathematical Genius, come in."

"I'm flattered, of course, but—"

"Take him away, Harry," Daisy said, making an imperious gesture. "Lock him in the bathroom for the night, and guard the door."

"But—"

"Come on, you." Harry dragged Cal to the bathroom, flung him in, and turned the key on him.

There were no windows. Cal walked up and down, thinking, examining fixtures, waiting for the others to get to sleep. Then he got down and whispered at the keyhole.

"Harry! Sssst! Why not let me out of here? Do me a favour, will you?"

Harry laughed, one hoarse bark. "Do *you* a favour? That's really rich. After all you've done to me."

"Look, Harry, I'm sorry about—"

"Oh, don't get me wrong. I don't care about Mary Junes any more. Not at all. I forgot all about her. I mean, there's plenty other cookies in the jar. But—do *you* a favour! That's really rich."

Cal curled up in the tub and tried to sleep. From time to time, Harry emitted another strangled bark. "Boy! That really is rich. Do *him* a favour!"

In the morning the five of them started out for Las Vegas. Cal's blindfold was left off, and he was able to see that the motel in which he'd spent the night was right across the street from *The El Cantina Bar*.

While he nursed his hangover, the other four began a spirited conversation about the nature of the universe, as perceived through the working of coincidence.

Daisy maintained that in coincidence we see no other hand but the Deity's. She related numerous instances of simultaneous birthdays, albinism, people's being struck by lightning or meteors, and the odd results of Dr. Rhine's experiments.

Jack owned she had a point. Harry agreed that coincidences did seem to happen.

Brian Gallopini replied that it would be blasphemy to blame the Deity for mine cave-ins, for midair plane crashes maiming children, for widows losing their compensation cheques.

Harry clung to the notion that accidents would happen.

Daisy pointed to the fiction of the eighteenth century. She cited coincidences in *Tom Jones* and *Humphrey Clinker*. If such were the work of authors (Fielding and Smollet), why could not coincidences in Life have an Author (God)?

"By thunder!" Brian swore. "Are you trying to tell me, woman, that you and I are naught but puppets, jerked about at the whim of some buffoon of a novelist? Pish! You may believe as you please, but know you that I am a free agent. I command my hand to move; it moves. See?" He demonstrated.

Daisy laughed. "Only because you were destined to command it to move. You were commanded by the Author of All."

But the Professor lapsed into a moody silence and would not answer. Some of the taller buildings and larger signs of Las Vegas were coming into view.

Offering Cal a pinch of Bergamot snuff, the Professor then began to explain to him his own ingenious betting system.

"Each time the bettor loses a bet," he said earnestly, "he doubles his next bet. Since every run of luck must needs obey the immutable laws of Destiny, the first winning bet must needs more than make up for all his previous losses at one stroke!"

Cal groaned inwardly, but said nothing, reminding himself that he was a guest—and a prisoner.

"It is a complex system, but foolproof, as you can see," concluded Gallopini. "Yet it shews forth the orderly working of the universe. And the universe *is* orderly. To say it is not is to believe in magic. One might as well say that the man in that sign could go walking across the desert."

The sign he indicated was a giant representation of a prospector atop one casino. In one hand he held a pan of nuggets, while the other moved up and down, as if beckoning. It was one of the more famous signs of the city, and could be seen for miles at night.

Now, as the horrified group watched, it did seem to take a step. Daisy screamed, a rich baritone scream, while the professor went as white as a periwig.

"Ah, it is all right. It is only falling. Perhaps being demolished," he said. They watched the sign buckle and disintegrate with some relief. An upsetting coincidence, but not supernatural. The others relaxed, but Cal remained rigid, still staring at the skyline.

"I think I know what this is all about," he breathed. In the distance another sign tumbled, as little grey boxes swarmed over it like ants. "We'd better turn around and head the other way at once."

"Don't be an ass," said the Professor. "I've come here to make my fortune, and demme, I'm not turning around on your command. Hold your tongue, sir!"

"Turn around! Please!" Cal said to Harry, who was driving.

"As a favour to you, I suppose," he sneered.

"Listen. There is something loose in that city—a secret weapon —and it's out of control. I don't know how it got here, but it looks like it has taken over Las Vegas. I'm sure of it. Believe me, our lives are in danger if we enter the city."

"Stuff and nonsense!" snapped the Professor. "I do *not* believe you, sir. But—so that I cannot be accused of being unfair—we might stop at a telephone and call ahead. We could reserve rooms at the same time that we prove your nonsensical theory has no foundation. Stop at that phone ahead, Harry. Stop, I say!"

But the car continued on past the phone. In fact, it picked up speed. "I can't control it," said Harry. "It's like something has hold of it. The steering is locked, and there's some kind of—cable thing—reeling us in."

They were close enough to the city to see destruction, now, and swarms of boxy shapes moving over the broken faces of buildings and signs.

"What shall we do?" Daisy screamed.

"There is nothing we can do," said her fiancé quietly, tapping on the lid of his snuffbox. "It seems as if we shall go on accelerating until we hit something and probably die. *You* may prepare to meet *your* Author, my dear. Now, since we have perhaps a minute or two, I suggest that Mr. Potter tell us more about this fascinating machine."

CHAPTER X

CALLING DR. SMILAX

"Let us, however, look more closely at the facts."
A. J. AYER

SHORTLY BEFORE HE was to address the Joint Chiefs of Staff, Dr. Smilax stepped into the men's room adjoining the NORAD conference room and began briskly combing his hair. On such occasions, tension seemed to tighten his scalp and make it itch furiously, unless he could give it a quick, vigorous raking.

It was black, luxuriant hair shot with silver grey of the same shade as his foulard tie. This was embroidered with black anthrax bacilli, carefully knotted, and clipped with a tiny silver scalpel. His suit was a quiet grey, his shirt of television blue, though he had no real intention of appearing before news cameras. The only real spot of colour about him was his lapel pin from the Blood Bank, a red plastic droplet.

The bold outlines of Smilax's face were softened by a dapper moustache, while rimless glasses diluted the peculiar intensity of his gaze. Nevertheless his was the unrelenting expression of a man used to commanding, not acquiescing. He could not fawn, like most civilian "experts" consulted by the Joint Chiefs. Smilax gave orders, he did not beg to be given orders, and all the clerkliness in his appearance could not disguise the fact. Breeding, he thought, permitting himself a small, ironic smile, will out.

Toto Smilax, M.D., D.V.M.S., Ph.D. (Chem.) and M.E.E., was the scion of a good family, though only by accident. One of his earliest memories was of his mother's shaking her head and saying, "Son, I don't never want you to go wrong like I done."

He was five years old before he learned what "going wrong" meant; it meant having a child without being married first. At once Toto began to worry that he would, somehow, actually give birth to a child out of wedlock. Every morning he looked in his bed fearfully, to see if a baby had arrived.

Lotte Smilax, his mother, had never married. She often told little Toto how her father had been an important man in the

West, and how she had brought disgrace upon the family by allowing the mad butler to rape her at gunpoint.

"It was all because my Daddy never beat me," she would say. "Oh, if only he had beat me! But I mean to do better by you, my son. I won't make the same mistakes. I want to give you every chance I never had."

So saying, she would commence larruping him with anything handy: her boot, a whip, a ladle, or a belt.

School was for Toto equally onerous, for the other children tortured him without mercy, to the limits of their fiendish imaginations. They poked him with compasses, stole or tore his books, implied that his mother was a "hoor" and that he was born out of wedlock, stoned him, made up songs about him, and invited him to eat (in summer) sand and mud, and (in winter) unclean snow.

The reason they did all this was because, of course, his name was Toto. It was not a Christian name, it was not even the name of a famous hero, real or fictional. It was the name of a dog.

Poor Toto had been named for his mother's favourite character in fiction, Dorothy's little dog in *The Wizard of Oz*. Lotte, it must be confessed, was fond of animals, and her bookshelf was filled with dog books, including the complete works of Albert Payson Terhune and *Dog of Flanders*, which Lotte never read without weeping.

She may have been a stern disciplinarian, but Toto's mother was also a warm-hearted, impulsively generous creature, who never could resist bringing home a hungry dog or lame kitten. Generally the hearth was merry with one or two Lads, a Rex, a Spot, and perhaps half-a-dozen Snowballs and Midnights. Lotte often encouraged them to dine sitting up together at the table with her, for she loved to have company for dinner, and Toto for his own good was restricted to his bowl on the kitchen floor, marked with his name.

Every night, curled up in his little basket, Toto would hear his mother going out to her SPCA meeting. He would lay there and pray, naming each of her pets in connection with a different kind of painful death. To finish off the list, he would conjure up a set of slow agonies for Albert Payson Terhune, whom he somehow imagined to be Lotte's father.

One day they took one of the mangy Rexes to the Pet Clinic. Toto wandered around the building, discovering the mysteries of veterinary medicine. Through a glass partition he saw a cat undergoing Caesarian section to give up six kittens. Toto pressed his nose to the glass wistfully. It was all so beautiful—the bright red blood, the clean linen, the very mystery of reproduction itself, laid open by a glittering knife. So this was sex!

Within him, Toto's fierce little spirit rejected everything he had been taught. Having babies could not be so wrong after all. Nothing so solemn and bloody could be altogether bad. He vowed to become a vet.

When he was eight, the magic carpet of a court order removed him from his mother's custody and placed him with two kind, pleasant old maiden aunts in Dubuque. There were no more beatings, plenty to eat, a regular bed. There was a tutor instead of school.

From an illiterate child, unable to eat without lapping, Toto became a fine young gentleman, exceeding his aunts' wildest hopes in nobility and refinement. They spared no expense to teach him all modern and classical languages; under the best masters he learned mathematics, elocution, fencing and dancing.

Toto showed himself no mean scholar, becoming a vet at thirteen, and a physician and surgeon two years later. To keep his fingers supple for operating, he took up the violin, achieving a technical virtuosity that was remarkable. He seldom played, however, complaining the high notes hurt his ears.

In Zürich, Toto met a young English anaesthetist named Nan Richmons, and for the first time in his twenty years he knew a passion more overpowering than his devotion to science. Not only was Nan beautiful and intelligent, but her X-rays showed a crystalline symmetry that made his breath catch. How long would it be before he might gaze in reality upon that coil of colon, those ovaries, the perfect curves of her kidneys? How long before he might pluck that fragile bloom, her appendix? He asked Nan to marry him and become the subject of his surgical experiments, and—ah, peritoneal bliss untold!—she accepted.

The banns were published on two continents. Toto and Nan spent their evenings planning hysterectomies, new and dangerous techniques of anaesthesia. Then, without warning, their castles of aether collapsed.

A muffled stranger came to call upon Toto in his lab, where he was dissecting a cadaver on the eve of their wedding.

"You must not marry Nan Richmons."

"But why not?" asked Toto. His brow darkened. "I must warn you, sir, to be careful what you say about her."

75

"Why, you ask?" The stranger laughed savagely. "Two reasons: First, she is already married—to me."

"I care nothing about that. This is 1935, man! Let us be civilized. Her past is—"

"Stay! The second reason is—is that *I removed her appendix over two years ago.*"

Toto grew pale and staggered back a pace, laying a cadaverous hand to his palpitating heart. "Good God! Say that is a lie, you blackguard!" Sadly, the stranger shook his head.

"It is the truth."

"Then here." Toto snatched up a scalpel and offered it to him. "Remove my heart, sir, if you please. It is no longer of the slightest use to me."

The engagement was broken at once. Nan, despairing, took her life with a mixture of chloroform and nitrous oxide. Toto travelled then, to the Orient, to Africa and elsewhere, studying peculiar surgical techniques.

After the Second World War, he turned up in California, announcing his intention of starting a research laboratory. The Defence Department at once placed several million dollars at his disposal. Toto shut himself up for another decade, doing pain research, during which time he churned out interesting books and monographs (*Aesthetic Surgery*; *The Painful Way to Health;* and a book of child care, *Spare the Rod? Never!*). He studied and conquered new fields of inquiry at the same time: physics, biochemistry, astronomy, biophysics and arachnology, like so many stands of grain, fell to his keen scythe of a mind. In 196– his researches culminated in the invention of the DNA computer known as QUIDNAC.

The existence of this type of computer was not generally known, its principle of operation was a military secret, and its manufacture was understood only by Dr. Toto Smilax himself, who now entered the NORAD conference room.

The Chiefs of Staff were seated behind a large table of gunmetal grey, as far as possible from one another. At one end reared the thin angular frame of Air Force General Ickers, a quick, bird-like man with a shrill voice. Once a test pilot, he still retained a more or less happy-go-lucky attitude about everything but the dignity of his office.

At the opposite end sat a leaden mass of flesh bundled into the uniform of Admiral of the Navy. Because he had once commanded a sub—or rather, a series of subs, each of which managed to have an improbable but genuine accident as soon as he had taken command—he still wore a dirty white turtleneck pullover under his jacket. He managed a sneer now and then, but otherwise the expression on his bloated, drowned-corpse's face was of despair and apathy.

In the middle sat General of the Army R.M.S. ("Happy") Meany, whose face seemed to try its level best to imitate both the countenances of his contemporaries. He never looked towards Ickers without a confident grin or wink of camaraderie; never towards Nematode without a rueful, commiserating sigh.

At a smaller table some twenty feet away sat a WAF secretary. When Dr. Smilax entered, all were watching the progress of a battle on the Big Board. One half of it showed the green lines and blue grids of a topological map; the other displayed jerky televised glimpses of actual skirmishing.

A contingent of paratroops had been landed in Altoona. The evening was murky—moonless, Smilax remembered—and the images were jiggly and confused (Nematode insisted the enemy was jamming the works for reasons of their own; Ickers declared the reception was perfect as far as he was concerned). Now and then a squat, blocky shape hurtled out of the gloom, made a grab at some man's weapon, and vanished again.

"Some sojers!" snorted the admiral.

One paratrooper was hit, low, by what appeared to be a twisted sort of typewriter. He dropped his machine gun and fell, arms flailing.

"I knew it wouldn't work," said Nematode slowly, savouring his words. "But why should anyone listen to me? I'm only the Admiral." He laced his thick fingers together and studied their dirty nails.

"One man knocked down doesn't mean a lost battle," snapped Ickers. His head bobbed, shaking silver plumage in emphasis. "Got the wind knocked out of him, that's all. He's playin' possum, so he can trick the enemy."

At that moment, the screen went dark. "I knew it!" crowed the admiral. "Now that thing has captured the camera."

"The hell it did!"

"Yup, captured the whole goddamned town, and our boys with it. Tonight Altoona—tomorrow the world! This'll be the end of civilization—and good riddance, I say!"

"What?" Ickers screeched. "How can you wear the uniform of

your country and say a rotten thing like that? That's a lie! Our United States will last a thousand years!"

"Well there's much to be said for both viewpoints," said General Meany. "Why don't we hear a few words from our expert on the matter, eh? Doctor, won't you tell us a little about this gadget of yours?"

" 'Gadget'? A trivial word for something to which I am sure you attach a great deal of importance, gentlemen. Oh—," he permitted himself a wry, professional smile as he rose and strolled to the blackboard—"I know I'm indulging in a semantic quibble, but we men of science are rather narrow about our definitions."

Taking chalk from his pocket, he wrote "Nomenclature: THE REPRODUCTIVE SYSTEM," across the top of the board. The three men pulled pads towards them and readied pens. Meany wrote "syst." and underlined it three times.

"The Reproductive System is composed of what we call *cells*." The doctor wrote it on the board. "The first cells were constructed at Project 32, as you all know. They were of a variety of types, differing from one another in two respects:

"(1) *Differing means of perception and communication*. These included metal detectors, radiation detectors, radar, cathode tubes, microphones, light pens, graphic inputs and displays, and typewriters. Only the first two of these were standard on all cells built.

"(2) *Differing modes of propulsion*. These included gear-driven wheels, jointed insectoid legs, rockets, propellors, and the inertial, or 'falling-cat' system. Just as a cat can right itself while in midair, so an object may be propelled by displacing weight 'outwards and backwards' rapidly. It moves as does a child scooting along in a cardboard box. We saw a soldier on television doing the same thing unconsciously—threshing his arms to restore his balance."

"Yes," chuckled the admiral, who was not taking notes. "We saw how well it worked for *him*, didn't we? He's only dead, that's all."

Ickers jumped up. "It's a glorious and fine thing to die in the service of our country," he shouted. "I only wish *everyone* had the chance to do so, right this minute!"

"Now gentlemen," said Meany. "Let's try to reconcile our differences. There is much truth in what each of you say. Perhaps the doctor would be good enough to give us his view on the matter?"

"How about a little action!" shouted Ickers. Meany filled in the single word on his pad with geometric forms. Nematode began drawing female genitalia. "Let's not sit around here all day. I want to get out there and *slam that thing in the gut.* My boy Grawk is out in the hall now, waiting for orders. Let's go-go-go!"

Dr. Smilax drew a cross-section of an individual cell. "The size varies," he explained, "for various hereditary and environmental reasons. The original cells were not of a size, and their differences have become in some cases quite marked. The armoured exterior of each cell is usually weatherproofed by paint, rubber or plastic coatings and the like. Apertures are maintained, through which tools can be projected: hooks, claws, cutters, welding equipment, etc. On some types the casing is expandable. In most types it can be opened to admit materials—or emit a neophyte cell.

"The space just inside the cell is where reproduction and maintenance take place. Manufacturing is quite limited in scope, consisting chiefly in adapting found objects to makeshift purposes.

"Templates for both mechanical and electronic components (such as integrated circuits) are constructed at the orders of the QUIDNAC control unit. All bearings and other parts requiring close tolerances are made by sintering; finer machining is done with acids.

"Any power supply may be used, if either it can be modified to fit into the cell or the cell can make sufficient modifications upon itself. We predicted, for example, that cells would be able to glue themselves to locomotives and take power from them, and I understand our prediction was correct.

"Now for the 'yolk' of our 'egg'," he said, with another dry, professorial smile, and pointed to the centre of his chalk diagram. "This is the QUIDNAC control unit, in three sections: (1) The DNA section; (2) the amplifying and interpreting section; and (3) the control linkage.

"The DNA section is a complex, compact means of storing and retrieving information. In it are stored about 10^{10}, or ten billion messages, many of them only three units long, but some as long as a million units. The fourteen simplest messages correspond to the rules of logic, to arithmetic computation, or to the mechanics of handling other data."

He wrote:

Message	Meaning	Conventional Symbol
AAA	"Either ... or ... or both"	$\vee$
CCC	"If ... then ..."	$\supset$
GGG	"... and ..."	$\cdot$
TTT	"... is equivalent to ..."	$\equiv$
GAGGAG	"zero"	o
GCGGCG	"positive"	+
GTGGTG	"negative"	—
TGTTGT	"... is identical with ..."	=
AGAAGA	"Record ..."	(Remember)
ATAATA	"Erase ..."	(Forget)
CGCCGC	"Duplicate ..."	(Repeat; Copy)
CTCCTC	"Transit ..."	(Tell me)

"These messages are encoded in a double helix of DNA. They are activated only by the appropriate input. In one sense, the QUIDNAC is completely programmed, since it is true that every message output, or response, has been encoded into the molecule of DNA. But different *sets*, different combinations of responses are not predictable, if only because of their very, very, varied variety." Again the smile, and again no response from his audience. "The total number of message combinations possible is equal to the sum of the squares of all the numbers from 1 to 10^{10}.

"All input data, or stimuli, are automatically recorded, and compared with previous stimuli. If they correspond, they are dealt with as in past successes; if they do not, various analogies are devised from past experiences. If no analogies seem to have the slightest relevance to the new stimuli, random responses are selected and tested. In effect, QUIDNAC learns, and as it learns *it alters the structure of the DNA molecule*. Alterations generally consist in breaking the molecule apart and reassembling it in new patterns, much in the manner of making anagrams from long words:"

Here he wrote: "JOHN THOMAS SLADEK"

And under it: "DNA'S MOL HATH JOKES"

"You see, a *mol* is a gram molecular weight, or the molecular weight of a substance expressed in grams. The molecular weight of our DNA is about 287×10^{16}, so the joke of it is that one mol would weigh about three trillion tons."

He laughed heartily at DNA's subtle jest. The three faces before him, however, remained fixed in their gargoyle patterns of joy, despair and indecision. Dr. Smilax cleared his throat and prepared to resume.

"British trillion or American trillion?" asked the WAF secretary. "Long tons or short tons?"

"I'll go into it later, if you'll make a note of it." A muscle in the doctor's scalp began twitching. "Now then:

"The second stage of the QUIDNAC control unit consists of a system of integrated circuits which translate and amplify the output of the DNA section. The third section consists of actual control mechanisms, switches, relays, etc., operating various 'limbs', 'organs' and functions of the cell. Tuned circuits are employed, so that a rather complex signal may be sent as an excitation 'clang', out of which each receiver selects its own signal. Our own nervous system works on much the same principle."

"What we'd like to know, Doctor," said the Army head, glancing nervously towards both ends of the table, "and I think I can safely say I speak for my colleagues here in this—what we'd like to know is, what does the QUIDNAC computer *look like*, and how can we shut it off?"

"The entire control unit looks much like a transistor radio," said the doctor. "The bulk of it is control linkage, however. The amplifying section is about the size of a lady's wrist watch. The DNA memory file is, of course, invisible. Its casing may be seen— it is roughly the size and shape of a light pencil dot."

"The US Air Force isn't likely to have much trouble slaughtering a few pencil dots," said Ickers, beaming.

"Well—" Smilax began, then sighed.

The admiral emitted a pained snort, his equivalent of a laugh. "I guess that finishes us," he said. "I always knew the human race was bound to be finished off by something like a bunch of pencil dots. It figures."

"Perhaps we're beaten," cajoled General Meany, "and perhaps again we have a chance. I think it's too early to tell, at this stage of the game. I defer judgement until we hear from our expert here."

"Are you trying to tell me," asked Ickers, "that in only a few days these invisible bugs have piled up enough junk to cover twenty thousand square miles? And we can't stop this?"

"I'm afraid that is correct," said Smilax, "though rather pessimistic. They have worked underground for over two weeks, preparing for this takeover. Moreover, they have only fenced, or enclosed, rather than covered the area, and I believe it to be only about 17,213 square miles. That you have had no success thus far in stopping it is evident," he added, with his eyes downcast. "That is why you have sent for me. I do foresee one way of stopping the Reproductive System—though you may find my way repugnant."

"I knew we weren't beaten!" screeched the Air Force head, and gave an exultant laugh. "What *is* your idea, doctor?"

"Sure, go ahead. What have we got to lose now?" said the admiral. "The human race is a dead letter, now."

Smilax lighted a display map. "The System seems to have three centres of growth, at the moment, and it is fencing off and surrounding the area between them. They are the lab at Millford, Utah; Altoona, Nevada; and Las Vegas. The judicious detonation of three thermonuclear devices of the order of 150 megatons each would, I feel confident, completely neutralize the System at these points. The remainder would be a simple matter of—I believe the expression is 'mopping up'—using smaller thermonuclear devices. I know what question you are going to raise in advance, so let me say I estimate the total number of civilian casualties at no more than a million."

"Did he say a million or a billion?" murmured the WAF.

"If it's the cost of our commitment," said the smiling Ickers, "I'm all for it!"

"That's about the population of Nevada and Utah combined," Admiral Nematode pointed out. "And this is election year. We'll never get Congress to buy the idea of bombing hell out of two states. Might as well throw in the sponge now."

"My colleagues both have a valid point," said Meany carefully. "Have you any alternatives, doctor?"

"Only a plan for a new line of research towards altering the System genetically. It has, fortunately or unfortunately, the ability to pass along acquired characteristics. Given about two months, we could—"

"Two months!" Nematode shouted. "In two months, it'll be covering the globe."

"No, by my estimate, if it grows at the present rate, it would reach 88 times its present size in eight weeks. It would then cover most of 1,514,788 square miles, that is, roughly the size of fifteen of our westernmost states, not including Texas or Oklahoma, but with the area of Maine thrown in."

82

"Oh, Christ."

Ickers had called in Grawk and seemed to be in a furiously jubilant state over what his subordinate was whispering to him. "Great! Great! Great! Tell them about it."

"I know this sounds like kind of a crazy idea," said the ugly little general. "But maybe it's just the kind of wacky thing that would work. Give a listen: I remember once in an old science fiction movie they got rid of the monster by electrocuting him. Remember that? Well we could try the same thing—just hook up the high voltage and juice it to death!"

"Science fiction," snorted the admiral.

"I think he has something," said Smilax. "It *may* work—by shorting out the fine circuitry—but if it fails, we gain nothing."

"At least we lose nothing," shrilled Ickers. Clapping Grawk on the back, he bawled, "Your idea, my boy. You're in charge. Tap the power line at Altoona. Get to work on it right away. Thumbs up."

"And when you fail," said the admiral with bilious charm, "it'll be thumbs up for you, all right. You'll be Airman Third Class Grawk—if we don't shoot you."

Meany summed it up. "Godspeed, Grawk," he said. "We wish you success and warn you not to fail."

"I ain't worried." Grawk carried his yellow grin and black cigar out of the door.

Another camera had been set up at Altoona, and now, Smilax having been invited to join the Joint Chiefs in their weekly game of Go-to-the-Dump, the four watched the new scene on the Big Board. A group of young people were parading in front of the barbed-wire barrier which the military had thrown up around the city. They carried signs saying: "WHAT HAPPENED TO ALTOONA?" "DOWN WITH DOOMSDAY" and "GIVE US BACK OUR WORLD".

"They'll find out soon enough what happened to Altoona," said the Army head, dealing. "If Grawk's plan comes off, and we get the thing on the run, we'll 'leak' the story tomorrow, through our usual reliable sources."

One girl seemed to be in the wrong parade. She wore white boots, and carried a sign saying: "GO GO GOPHERS!"

Then she turned, and Smilax could see another message hastily lettered on the back of the sign: "END OF THE WORLD UNFAIR TO YOUTH!"

A platoon of soldiers arrived, surrounded the protestors and began dragging them away.

83

"Where are they taking them?" Smilax asked General Meany.

"We'll keep them locked up until tomorrow night, or whenever this blows over. Why?"

"It's that girl in the boots, She seems a perfect subject for my latest pain experiments. I wonder . . ."

"I get it," said Meany, and nudged him. "Haha, I get it. Of course I'll have her seized for you. Where do you want her? Here?"

"Yes, I've set up in the infirmary. Thank you."

"Haha, you old scoundrel!"

"You don't know the half of it," said Smilax, gazing up at the girl—the image of Nan Richmons. He was already picturing the perfect symmetry of her kidneys.

CHAPTER XI

BEELE OF THE CIA

"Pause there, Morocco."
SHAKSPEARE

SUGGS KILLED TIME while waiting for his new partner by writing another postcard to his wife. He chose one which depicted the snake charmers in the market at Dar El Fna. "Dear Madge," he wrote, after some deliberation. "Still having wonderful time, though I miss you and Susie. Love, Bubby."

He wondered if he ought to say something about the insurance game being slow in Marrakech—insurance was his cover story—but decided against it. Madge probably thought he was just living it up with harem girls anyway. And so he would have been, if Suggs had not been terrified of disease. He remembered only too well the CIA training films of tertiary syphilis and advanced gonorrhea. . . .

A rumbling in his stomach reminded Suggs the Near East held other diseases for the unwary. He wished now he had brought along his own supply of food. Today Suggs had made fifteen trips to the bathroom, scoring them off with a kind of grim satisfaction in his journal.

He was not sure which of the descending passengers would be the new man, but he finally settled on the skinny young man in the eyeshade, who was shaking off a pack of urchins.

"You Green?" Suggs breathed, drifting past him.

"Huh?"

Suggs drifted past again. "You Mr. Green?"

"Oh, you must be Mr. Gray."

"That's right. Only my friends call me Suggs. B. Suggs. Why the eyeshade?" Suggs turned to confront his new partner openly. "What's your cover story? I guess you could say you're a sheep rancher, come to look over some rare breeding stock."

"My name is really Beele, Barthemo Beele. I'm under your orders, Mr. Suggs, but—"

"Just Suggs, please."

"Suggs, I don't know what kind of corruption is going on in

this town, but I want to do my level best to put an end to it. Do you know what just happened? One of those *little kids* tried to sell me something I feel certain was a narcotic!"

Suggs picked up Beele's suitcase and motioned towards the shay. When they had settled into place he told the driver the name of their hotel and turned to his new agent with a bit of advice. "Don't pay any attention to these little packs of beggars. They go on all the time, trying to sell you their sisters, hashish, brothers, mothers, *kif*, and so on. You'll get used to it."

"Used to it! I hope not! It's a disgrace and a crime. Haven't they a truant officer around here? Those kids ought to be in school. I mean to find out what kind of crime bosses are at the bottom of this. But, as I say, you're in charge here—"

Suggs shook his head sharply and indicated the driver. They rode on, sizing one another up in silence, silence broken only by the clopping of the horse down a scenic avenue of tangerine trees, and by the sick growling from Suggs's abdomen.

Looking at the older man, Beele saw a sunburned, bullnecked man with short-clipped greying hair, regular, unmemorable features. Suggs looked to be about forty and a pipeline engineer, and there was nothing to mark him off from the ordinary run of men but his cold, lacklustre eyes and a thin white scar on his forehead. So this was what CIA men looked like, on the job!

He wondered how he himself would turn out in the Agency. Did it take brains, guts, curiosity and honesty? Barthemo had these in abundance—yet did he have the indefinable something which distinguishes the CIA agent from others?

When Barthemo Beele was two years old, he was trained to use a little potty stool that was kept in a cupboard with a hanging cloth in front of it. This little secret, with its aura of shame, interested him so keenly that he had to lift the cloth and look at it a dozen times a day. To this single episode, he later felt, all of his curiosity could be traced. For little "Themo" developed an unfortunate habit of lifting hanging cloths to peer under them. And after he had lifted the skirt of a visitor, a bishop's wife, "Themo" received his first sound whipping.

Yet, as if his motto were *Video, ergo sum,* Barthemo went on lifting hanging cloths and looking under them, and was unable to resist doing so. He would lift the corner of a table cloth and stare at the table's legs, fascinated, flushed with guilt and a strange pleasure he could not name.

He grew to a skinny, secretive kid, addicted to tattling, to forming, with friends, secret clubs, and to writing what he hoped were dirty words on fences: FUDGE, SHAME, ORGANISM, and especially LOVE. One day by chance he lifted a blanket and found a couple of organisms making love: his mother and a man not his father.

Barthemo hastened to tell his father, who thanked him for his information by spanking him and locking him in his room for a day. When he decided the boy had learned his lesson, the elder Beele relented and let him out—but on condition that he mind his own business. Barthemo actually did have a business at this time, which was selling information to the police. For nickles, dimes and quarters, he would tell them which members of which secret clubs were stealing bike tyres from gas stations and magazines from drugstores. Later, for larger sums, he told them about car thefts and burglaries. This continued well into high school, when his duties as a school reporter took up most of his free time. The police gave him a present of money when he left for college, and told him he was the "Best little stoolie we ever had".

Someday, he thought, as the shay rolled along Boulevard Mohammed V, someday he would write a book, a defence of police informers: *They Call Me Stoolie*. "Why is it," he would write, "that those who risk their lives exposing murderers, thieves, dope peddlers, and every crooked and vicious element of our society, that those who do their duty as citizens (for *not* to report a crime is misprision), are looked on by society with loathing and distaste?"

Looking at Beele, Suggs saw a skinny, nervous-looking young man on whom an eyeshade, with a press card in the band, seemed a needless affectation. Suggs amused himself by imagining better cover stories for Beele. In a neat, dark suit, with an attache case, he could pass for an IBM salesman, perhaps. Or he could have grown a beard and looked like one of them Peace Corps freaks— buncha Commie fanatics. Fanaticism, that was it: the old-young look he had, the coldness in his face and a pinch of the true fanatic, summed Beele up for him. He wondered what it would take to make Beele kill a man. The kid might make a passable killer, with the proper instruction from Suggs—maybe too good a killer. Suggs wondered how long it would be before he would have to kill Beele.

"By the way," he said. "Try not to eat anything or drink the water here. I'm trying to get in a consignment of American food and water. The stuff here is murder."

"The runs?"

As if in answer, Suggs's stomach growled. Only it was not his stomach, he realized, but Beele's.

The younger man nodded glumly. "Yup, I got 'em, too. Must have been that Denver sandwich and cup of Boston coffee I had before I left the States."

While Beele signed the register and filled out the police form at the hotel desk, Suggs wrote on a picture postcard of the snake-charmers at Dar El Fna, "Dear Madge. Still having wonderful time, though I miss you and Susie. Love, Bubby." He handed it to the smiling clerk and received in exchange his room key and a thick airmail letter. It was from Madge's lawyer's office. There was no need to open it.

"It's not fair!" he whispered, crushing the letter into his pocket. "To dump a divorce on me *now*, of all times! Well, I just don't have time to worry about it, that's all." Nevertheless, he bit his lip, thinking of the possible effects this might have on his career. In the Agency, men with marital problems were passed over for promotion.

In the room, Beele relaxed on a settee while Suggs paced back and forth, explaining the mission. He took up a long, curved knife and toyed with it as he spoke.

"The French are launching a new missile from somewhere in the vicinity—we don't know where yet. They call it *Le Bateau Ivre*, and I've found out the name of the astronaut—young French Air Force pilot named Marcel Brioche. It cost me one of my best men to find out that little piece of information." His guts growled with scalding pain, and Suggs began to pace like a caged animal.

"I know the shot will take place soon, but I don't know where in the environs of Marrakech they're stashing the ship. Our first objective, therefore, will be to find out the date and precise point of launching.

"They have two reasons for hiding it. First," he pared one fingernail with the knife, "they have some new super-fuel, better than anything we've come up with so far. We want it, so does Russia. Only we want it worse, and I'll tell you why. This stuff is so hot, the only kind of exhaust nozzle they can use is made out of a material called reuttite. And the world's supply of reuttite is—"

88

"In Nevada!" Beele exclaimed. Then, thinking of the bright boxes of the day before, he wondered if the reuttite still were in Nevada. "They used to make gas mantles out of it, and—"

"Yeah, yeah, I see you been briefed on that already. Well, the French have been secretly buying up old gas mantles for years, preparing for this *coup*.

"Which brings us to their second reason for hiding the mission." He decapitated another nail. "We think they may try to actually put a man on the moon. That means they could *claim* the whole works—with nasty consequences for the rest of the world. See what I mean?"

The kid looked thoughtful. "No, I guess I don't see," he admitted.

Suggs snarled, "What's the matter, you dense or something? France on the moon means more than just a tricolor on the Mare Nubium. It'll mean French control of the Earth! How'd you like to be a slave of the French Republic, eh? Imagine what *that* would be like: All the restaurants stunk up with garlic and all the roads choked up with crummy little cars. They'd make you eat *snails* instead of decent food (like a steak and french fries). You couldn't even get a coke anymore—they'd make you drink their rotten *wine*! Fairy art museums! Lousy beer! VD! Crumbly cigarettes! No men's deodorants!"

He wheeled and flung the knife at the door. Despite its awkward shape, the blade spun end-over-end neatly and caught, quivering. "That's what I think of Frogs!" he grated.

"What are we supposed to do, stop the moon shot?" Beele asked, when he dared breathe.

"Only as a last resort. There's another way, I think. The rocket they designed is supposed to have a two-man capsule, but only one Frenchy is going along. Now we've got to persuade him to take one of us along with him, so we can 'study the effects of the new fuel', but also so we can counter-claim the moon. The trouble is, the Russians are trying to do the same thing. There are two of them in town, Vovov and Vetch.

"It should be easy to persuade him to throw in his lot with us, rather than them," opined Beele. "I don't see how he could quibble, when it's a matter of choosing between democracy and totalitarian slavery."

"Yeah, yeah, and the chief OK'd a voucher for a quarter million dirham, too," said Suggs, thoughtfully. "That's fifty grand. I hope Moscow can't go higher."

"A bribe? You're going to offer him *a bribe*?"

Suggs stared at his new assistant incredulously, wondering if he could possibly be as naïve as all that. His meditations were only broken into by an urgent, scalding message from his intestines.

That evening they went to a small motel on the edge of town overlooking the Atlas Mountains to see Marcel Brioche. He proved to be a personable young man with handsome, immobile features, wearing a dress uniform of the French Air Force. A look of surprise and annoyance flickered across his face, then he smiled.

"Good evening, Monsieur Suggs," he said. "I was just going out to dinner. What is it you wished to see me about?" He spoke standing in the doorway, and did not ask them in.

"If you know my name, maybe you know my game," Suggs snapped.

"Please, please. I have no time to fence. At any moment, my friends will be here—"

"I'll be brief, Brioche. We represent the US government, as you know already, no doubt. We are prepared to deal—"

"I am not. *Bon soir.*"

"Wait. All we ask is that you take one of our men with you, as an observer. We have no intention of interfering with your moon shot—if you cooperate with us. The ship, we know, will hold two men. What harm can it do to take along—an *autostoppeur*?"

"A hitchhiker? Let us speak in English, if you please; in very plain English. You ask me why I am not anxious to cooperate with your government. Very well, I will tell you.

"When I first heard of *Le Bateau Ivre*, three years ago, I was engaged to be married. The ship was planned to take the two of us on a honeymoon. But two years ago, when work on the ship had progressed too far to be cancelled, she left me."

"My sympathies," said Barthemo Beele. "I can understand how you feel. My wife has just left me, too."

"Oddly enough, I'm being served with divorce papers right now myself," chuckled Suggs. "But that's the breaks. Why didn't you get another girl?"

"Let me tell you what happened. The man she left me for was an American Air Force liaison officer at NATO in Paris. He had a brief affair with her and then dropped her. Liaison officer—*drôle*, eh? He had a brief *liaison* with her, you see?" There were tears in the astronaut's eyes. He was not weeping, however, but smiling dangerously. "She threw herself from the Eiffel Tower.

You ask me why I have not replaced her? The answer is obvious, I should think. No one can ever replace her. Ah, there are my friends now."

He indicated a taxi drawing up before the motel. In it were Vetch and Vovov. Brioche drew on his white gloves.

"You don't understand!" Beele said passionately. "We free nations must cooperate in space, not compete. We have to pull together to beat totalitarian Russia."

"I would suppose space big enough to hold all three mighty nations," the Frenchman murmured with a mild salute.

"How does two hundred fifty thousand dirham sound, Brioche?" asked Suggs desperately.

"You do not insult me only because I understand how it is with you Americans. You wish always to purchase the honour of others. That is because, of course, you have none of your own. *Bonsoir, messieurs.*"

With a careless wave he strode away, leaving his door unlocked. "You haven't heard the last of this!" Suggs screamed after him. The two Russian agents grinned hugely as their taxi accepted its third passenger.

"See you round, Suggs," Vovov called out, making an obscene gesture.

Vetch, a small man with a scholar's beard and a thoughtful manner, kept quiet and let Vovov do the talking. Vovov could always talk, joyfully and persuasively, even when his mouth was full, as it was now, of toast and caviare. He spoke English, as Brioche insisted.

"Caviare and champagne!" Vovov crowed. "Caviare and champagne! The one from the icy bowels of the Baltic sturgeon, the other from the pale, temperate, shady hills of France. They go together like France and Russia go together. Each is perfect in its own right, yet the combination, it is—" As words failed him, he seized another slice of warm toast and spread it with caviare.

"The Americans," he said, cramming his mouth full and choking slightly. He coughed, masticated and swilled champagne for a moment, then continued speaking through his food. "The Americanff are pigff! Pigff!"

"Eh?" The astronaut was not really paying attention, but letting his own champagne go flat. He had already had too much to drink, and, as always, it plunged him into gloomy thoughts of the one person he ought to be having champagne with.

"Fwine! They are—excuse me—swine!" said Vovov.

"Swine? Yes, that is exactly it." Brioche thought of the man who had taken her life—the swine named General Grawk.

The alert waiter, proud of his minimal English, brought them more champagne. *"Encore bouteille de swine, messieurs?"* He poured it before they could refuse.

"The Americans have no love," Vovov went on. "Only supermarkets and superhighways. Factories and mass living. Faugh!" He sprayed roe. "What is their art? Comic books. Negro work songs, stolen and sung by white exploiters. Western movies. They were not content with murdering off the poor Indian, no, they must *glorify* that murder. Again and again, he must fall off that pony, to satisfy the bloodlust of the decadant imperialists. Bah! I remember one film—*Battle of Comanche Arroyo,* it was called —where they showed the *same* strip of film over and over again, depicting an Indian falling off his pony dead. They hoped their depraved audience would not notice."

"Was that with John Wayne?" Brioche asked, interested.

"No, I believe it was—I forget who. But you know, it was the one where the colonel wants them to stay and hold the fort, but the captain—the young one who's really in love with the colonel's wife?—Well, he—"

"Oui, oui, je—I remember it very well!" exclaimed the astronaut. "And then the captain is going to take a squad out to Comanche Arroyo, even though he knows it's certain death, they'll be massacred, because he knows he can gain the fort enough time to send for help!"

"Remember his last words?" Vovov began to weep as he poured another round of champagne. " 'It is a far, far better thing I do, than I have ever done, and it is a far, far better reward I go to, than I have ever known.' Ah, it wrings the heart even of a strong man, a speech like that."

"Ah yes. Wonderful film."

After several minutes of moody silence, Vetch spoke. "At the risk of spoiling our little Film Festival," he said drily, "I must ask you to get around to the real topic for discussion. That is, will you, Marcel Brioche, take a Russian observer along on your moon trip? We offer you no money, no material rewards— we'll leave that sort of behaviour to the Americans. No, all we can offer you is the knowledge that you are assisting in the toppling of imperialism and the glorious expropriation of the expropriators."

Brioche shook his head. "No, I cannot help you. I am for France, and for France alone. The only person I ever wanted to take to the moon with me—is far, far beyond the moon now. I go alone."

He rose and in desolate silence took his departure.

In Russian, Vetch said, "I am afraid we are going to have to kill him. A pity he isn't working for the right side. An honest sort of chap."

He noticed that Vovov was staring before him, red-eyed, with a bleak expression on his face. Vetch nudged him.

"Don't take it so hard," he said. "Remember, we are agents. We cannot afford to make friends with our dinner companions, for the very reason that we might have to kill them. An agent has *no friends*. We must be prepared to sacrifice anyone—"

"Shhh!" said Vovov, his broad face puckered with annoyance. "I almost had it—the name of the actress who played the colonel's wife. Was it Virginia Mayo? No ..."

CHAPTER XII

OUR HEROINE

*"Of love as a spectacle, Bathsheba had a fair knowledge;
but of love subjectively she knew nothing."*

HARDY

AS AURORA LET the car coast to a stop, B476 scrambled up on the back of the seat and began to chatter, complaining of the cessation of motion.

"There, now," she said, but B476, a black-and-white laboratory rat, continued shivering nervously until Aurora caressed his back with her thumb.

Lighting a cigarette, she leaned back and gazed out at crooked telephone poles like the masts of becalmed ships. The masts were beginning to throw long shadows, now, and Aurora was lost.

She banged open the glove compartment door, then shut it at once. Reflex insisted on her looking there again for the Nevada roadmap, while she knew it was in the pocket of her raincoat, hanging up at home in Santa Filomena, several hundred miles away.

How many hundred, she had no idea. Clearly this road was becoming a cowpath, and it led north, not east. She had started out from Santa Filomena this morning, with the idea of reaching Millford by nightfall. It seemed that the last "DETOUR—NO ENTRY —MILITARIZED ZONE—DANGER" sign had pointed her off in the wrong direction. She could be a dozen or a hundred miles off the Utah highway now. There seemed to be nothing to do, however, but press on.

Sighing, she crushed out her cigarette in the already choked ashtray. Then she unclipped it and emptied it out of the window. Wind caught the plume of ash and whirled it away in streamers the sun made golden orange. Dust to dust, ashes to desert ash. Yucca Flats could not be far from here. A few motes remained, flying about her in senseless Brownian motion, flecks of fiery light.

> *Brightness falls from the air;*
> *Queens have died young and fair;*
> *Dust hath closed Helen's eye*

B476 and B893 had snuggled up close to her on the seat. Laboratory rats were always weak and prey to chills, and they were sensitive to this slight coolness as the sun fell. It was perverse of her, she thought, to be caring about the fate of a pair of sickly rats when the human race was about to be strangled by its own invention. She was being...

Abnormal?

Of child prodigies, a magazine article once had said: "It is not true to suppose they cannot live happy, adjusted, fulfilled lives. The popular notions of neurotic 'quiz kids' just aren't true."

Aurora had been three years old when she read the article and pondered its promise. Was it so? Was she going to have a happy, fulfilled life? Was she, then, just the same as real people? Or was she going to be singled out, as her father was singled out, for special torment?

The latter was the truth, as she had known it was at three years old. To his face, they called her father Charlie, but behind his back, she knew, he was "that crazy inventor fella", and they laughed at him with a kind of fear in their eyes. As she would later see, it was the reason for the practical jokes. Not a trick was missed, from tipping his outhouse and hanging a toilet on the weathervane of his barn to more malicious fun like burning up his corncrib, full. He never seemed to grow angry, only perplexed. He would puff at his unlit, usually unfilled, pipe and survey the poisoned dog or the nail driven in the oil pan of his tractor as if it were a kind of equation that might be worked out by dint of hard concentration.

Now, as she put the car in gear and moved on up the dwindling road, it seemed almost as if someone were playing a practical joke on Aurora. Another DETOUR sign appeared, pointing off to a a pair of worn ruts that could not possibly lead anywhere. Shrugging, she obeyed.

B476 climbed up on her shoulder and, snuggling between her neck and the back of the seat, disposed himself for sleep. He and B893 could not be used for experiments. They were "leftovers", rats which, because of genetic defects or peculiar conditioning, were useless for behavioural experiments. She had developed a habit of picking up such and making pets of them for the few months they lived. True, they were sports, freaks, abnormals—but then Aurora knew how to empathize with abnormality.

Aurora was a genius, and in a community where genius was treated as a suspicious deviation from the norm. The campaniform symmetry of the normal distribution curve of IQ's at her first school had grown a hump like Gibraltar before they noticed her, and sent her to a "special school for exceptional children". Her classmates had cleft palates, cataracts, lustreless minds. It was somehow unclear to the teachers why Aurora was there; they suspected her of some hidden and therefore more horrible defect.

Aurora was not long at the special school. Studying at home, she took her high-school diploma by mail at ten years of age. At thirteen she graduated *summa cum laude* in behavioural psychology from the University of Minnesota, and at seventeen she became Associate Professor of Psychology at the University of California at Santa Filomena.

It was then she had assumed the plain and prudent appearance that now took the place of character in her professional life. She wore short-cropped hair (but not too short), short and lightly-tinted nails, and semi-sensible shoes. Besides the neat suit she now wore, there were five others in her closet at home, in varying shades of grey. She wore only enough makeup and enough jewellery to avoid being known as the kind of woman who uses none. It was not that Aurora (the real Aurora who resided some-where inside the professional figure) would not have liked to be admired, but her situation required special tact. She needed to look unappetizing to her male students (many of them older than herself), to keep them at a cool professional distance. She needed to look older for her colleagues, who despite themselves tended to be unconsciously sceptical of the efficiency of the very young. So it was that the disguise of the classroom and lab became a habit, in both senses of the word. She was twenty, felt twenty-five, acted like thirty, and was occasionally taken for thirty-five.

Two figures stood in the roadway on the left, apparently waiting for a ride in the direction she had come. Aurora slowed to ask them if they knew the way to Millford, Utah. When they turned around, Aurora was startled to recognize a pupil of hers, Kevin Mackintosh.

"What are you doing in Nevada, Mr. Mackintosh?" she asked, astonished.

The young man's eyes seemed glazed. Instead of answering, he nudged his companion. "We really *are* high, Ron," he muttered. "That chick over there looks like one of my profs."

"Oh, that was real good stuff," the other assented, looking off in another direction. "What chick?"

Aurora grew a bit nervous. She shifted into first, and kept her foot on the clutch. "Have you any idea which way is the road to Utah?" she asked earnestly.

Kevin Mackintosh seemed not to be looking at anything. "The road to you-Tao," he breathed. "The seven-fold path. Look!" He flung up both arms to the sunset. "Apocalypse! The wise virgins light their lamps! The black yoni of Night accepts the flaming lingam of Day!"

"Yeah, War of the Worlds," said Ron.

"Ma'am, my buddy Ron here and I have seen Hell itself. We have seen the death of the world, in flaming technicolour. Paratroops fighting to the death with Puppet People. They arrested our friends, but we got away."

"Who did?" she asked. "The Puppet People?"

"No, the Paratroople People. The Army. It's the end of civilization."

"Repent!" screamed the other. "Did you see *Gorgo*?"

"My buddy here and I are making our way across the Sahara here without water even, and we're going to Morocco."

Aurora relaxed a bit, recognizing in them a couple of not-too-bright kids from the college, dramatizing their first taste of pot. "If you're not particular which way you get there," she said crisply, "you can come along with me to—I hope—Utah."

"No thank you, ma'am. I mean really, we're going to Morocco; Ron's got his dad's airline credit cards. We've had it to here with this country. The real scene is Morocco, with Dorothy Lamour and Bing Crosby and Bob Hope and William Burroughs." He began to sing, off-key, an approximation of "The Road to Morocco".

"I dig," said his companion. "Did you see *Casablanca*?"

"If we ever get a ride out of here. There's nothing going by but jeeps and tanks, like in *Battleground*, and they don't stop."

"Thanks," said Aurora, and let out the clutch.

"Not thanks," Mackintosh explained patiently. "*Tanks*."

As she started driving off, Ron looked at her and screamed, "O my God, I'm coming down! O my God! THERE'S A RAT GROWING RIGHT OUT OF HER HEAD!"

"Yeah! Hey, Ron, you ever see *The Lost Weekend*?"

A sign informed her that the lights on the left were those of Piedport, Nevada, four miles off the road. As Aurora was about to heave a sigh of relief and take the turnoff—for at least Piedport would have a hotel—the town's lights went out. She stopped and waited for several minutes, but nothing happened. There was no use, as she saw it, stopping there, when she could as easily push on to a town at least equipped with lights.

The radio gave nothing but a squeal that excited B476. None of the pushbuttons seemed to have any effect other than changing the pitch of the whine. It was odd, because it could not be later than 9:00. There ought to be dozens of stations.

Manually she found a weak station in the southeast.

"... y'all keep them cards and letters comin', hear? Keep fahrin' 'em right at me, now, we appreciate hearin' from you, neighbours ... tunes you want ... Here's a wahr service bulletin, folks, seems like they had a little blackout over Calyforny way. Nevada, Calyforny, Oregon, Utah, Washington ... Iowa, Kansas..."

In the middle of its alarming list, the station faded into oblivion. She found a San Francisco station, then, but it only kept urging her not to call her power company.

"They are doing everything in their—I mean, everything possible to restore service. I'll just repeat the wire service bulletin with that message from the Pentagon: 'The blackout has been caused by a generating plant short in Nevada, following an experiment the full nature of which cannot be divulged, but which was vital to our national security. Power will be restored as soon as possible.' That was the Pentagon's message. Now, once again, *do not call* the power company...."

She began to see military vehicles parked along both sides of the road. Apparently they were abandoned, or the occupants were playing possum. Perhaps there was more to what Mackintosh & Company had said than she'd supposed. And the blackout...

She pulled off the road and parked. Knowing the potential danger of Project 32 was disturbing, but having the danger become actual was too horrible to understand at once. She needed to skirt the thought, she decided, switching off the lights. She needed to contemplate the calmness of the sky.

It was brighter than she had ever seen it, since the farm in Minnesota. There were no lights below to blot anything out, and she was stunned by the heavens' brilliance. There were Sirius and Aldebaran, pointing to the Pleiades, Orion between them. There were Castor and Pollux. She thought once more of the nights when she had learned their names, peering through one of her father's cracked, unusable telescopes.

At this time of year the farm would smell of corn and creak

with crickets—as it did through nearly three seasons of the year. Unperiodically, through the night, the farm's only "livestock", the Rooster, would crow. Any time was dawn to the Rooster; he was like the broken clock on the mantel and the broken clock in the hall. Periodically, her father had set out to fix one of the clocks, but she never heard one of them tick.

He invented a chicken-skinning machine, but somehow hadn't the heart to try it out on the Rooster, or indeed any chicken. So, though it was a fine-looking implement, they both agreed, it stood out on the lawn, becoming finally a rusty fixture, a perch for the Rooster when he announced the 11 p.m. dawn.

On the lawn were scattered further ornaments and perches as the years went by—A hot air balloon that leaked. A kind of mechanical birdbath shower which birds avoided. An improved kind of sewing machine. And about 168 telescopes, the first begun at Aurora's birth, that is, at her mother's death, the last left uncompleted seventeen years later.

Each time, he would grind lenses diligently for a day or two, then veer off into some other project. Of all the telescopes in the yard, the only one which worked was one he'd bought at a rummage sale and repaired with scotch tape. Through it Aurora had squinted at the Square of Pegasus, Vega and Cassiopeia's chair, the same unchangeable stars she now looked at out the windshield.

A black, hideous shape came between her and the stars. The car door opened and a thick-necked dwarf in uniform climbed in beside her. He left the door open for a moment, to look at her in the light.

"Keep cool, baby," he growled, waving a gun. "I'm General Grawk of the US Air Force, and I never raped a lady in my life. Never had to, if you get my meaning. Course there's always a first time, ain't there? Haha."

"What do you mean by this? Get out of my car!" She said it in her most severe schoolmarm voice. He chuckled.

"I'm commandeering this car, lady. National emergency. Maybe you heard about the big power failure?" He thumbed his chest. "I did that. Anyway, I need a car and driver, and you're elected." He moved over a bit closer. "It don't have to be all *that* bad, you know."

A faint squeal sounded from under the general.

"Get up! You're sitting on my pet rat!" she shrieked.

An instantaneous transformation took place. One moment he was a confident, grinning, aggressive little ape; the next he was screaming and vaulting into the back seat. The body of B893 lay flattened on the seat cushion. Aurora picked it up by the tail. It was dead. A strange smile played across her features as she lifted it, turning in the light.

"RATgetthatRATawayfrommEgetitawayRAT!" he screamed.

"Get out of my car. Now."

The gunbarrel swept B893 out of her hand and out of the open door. Grawk climbed back into the front seat and looked at her with a changed—a more respectful—expression. "I like you," he said. "Pretty cool. Pet rat, eh? That was good. But let's get rolling, now. Turn right at the next milestone." He slammed the door. Aurora did not move.

"I have another pet rat in the car with me," she said coldly, savouring each word. "A *live* one."

"WHERE? O God, is it *on me*? Where?"

"I have it safely out of your reach, for the moment. But unless you throw your gun in the back seat and start behaving like a gentleman, I shall *stuff this rat down your collar!*"

"You—you're kidding." Long silence. "There couldn't be another—is there?" Another long silence, then the gun thudded into the back seat.

"Now, general, I'll drive you where you wish to go, if you'll tell me what this is all about."

"We'll head for NORAD HQ in Colorado. That's safest," he said in a shaken voice. "I can't tell you what I'm doing here—it's a secret."

"If it has anything to do with Project 32, you may tell me," said Aurora, and handed him her purse. "My identification is in there."

"Who are you?" He fumbled in the purse, held up a card and trained a penlight on it. "Aurora Candlewood, Ph.D., Special Psychological Consultant for Project 32. A young kid like you? What does the fancy title mean, kid?"

"If you are going to tell me what I think you are going to tell me, it means Project 32 needs me badly."

"I'll tell you what we need," he said. "We need a good dragon-slayer."

"Right. Now suppose you tell me a little more about the dragon?"

CHAPTER XIII

WONDERJOURNEY

"Rudis indigestaque moles"
OVID

As THE CAR picked up speed the conversation within slowed, until, by the time they were flying into the outskirts of the deserted city, the five had grown strangely silent.

The car swerved, slowed, bumped down steel rollers into an unlit tunnel. Cal felt it buffeted by blasts of steam and water; he could smell the suds. There was the scream of saws on steel, and the dead blackness popped and flashed with livid gleams. By their uncanny light, Cal saw he was alone. The four others, the car, everything familiar was gone but the third of the seat to which he was still safety-strapped, which moved forward on invisible tracks to some rendezvous of its own.

He crashed through double doors into a room full of blood-red light, full of well-dressed mute figures. Mannikins, he thought with relief. In the corners, naked mute limbs in charnel heaps. The upper half of a dummy, weakly upright, slid down an inclined oily countertop, cracking the wall with its face and falling back. A bell sounded distantly. Sprinklers drizzled on the non-existent fire, while delicate water-wheels revolved beneath them. In the atro-sanguinous shadow, the dummy's smashed face and nose-hole received the rain.

* * *

Brian Gallopini found himself inexplicably alone, as the seat to which he was fastened moved into dry yellow sunlight. Light blazed white-red on his retina; he squinted at the globes. Artificial suns? No, goldfish bowls, fishbowls of gold lofted on levers to the sun, a sun-offering. The goldfish floated belly-up.

* * *

Cats crawled along upper shelves, going from nowhere to no-where. A few of them wore gold or silver watches strapped about their middles. One paused, near enough for her to read the watch. It was wrong. Daisy saw the date change from 7 to 8 with a click.

The cat gave a tiny scream and moved faster. It was only then Daisy noticed it was pulling a little pie tin full of machine parts.

*　　*　　*

Dipterous toy helicopters roamed the room, weaving fine copper wire in peculiar, meaningless patterns. Jack yawned.

*　　*　　*

Every can seemed to have rusted enough to admit a few bacteria. The buildup of gas was terrific, as Harry gladly demonstrated. He plunged his knife into a can that exploded black juice over his hand. He laughed.

"Sauerkraut!" he said. "Rotten sauerkraut!"

Cal did not laugh. "It's odd. Most of the stock is gone, and the rest is rotten. In only a few days. Mysterious. Is there anything left?"

Harry laughed again. "Nothing to write home about," he said, plunging his knife into another can. It squittered black and grey curds.

Later Cal would see how the system incorporated these exploding cans into a sort of "internal combustion" engine, using an old auto cylinder block, reloading eight cans after every revolution. But just now he was watching the shopping carts.

*　　*　　*

Ferriferous were the stately wheels of the sumptuous "ironclad", or locomotive, which stood upon rails of ferric metal, burnished bright. It looked powerful, and appearances, in this case, were not deceiving, for it fairly chuffed with impatience to be off. Steam issued forth and hissed insistence into the ironic fists, then the behemoth moved down inclined grooves towards an enormous loop-the-loop. Roaring up to 110 miles per hour, the leviathan looped and looped again. Switched into the vertical circle ($\frac{1}{4}$ mile high), it would continue thus until it "ran out of steam", as it were.

Jack watched the engine, awaiting its fall. Its blue-green lights, the colour of *Calliphoridae*, shone in the afternoon haze. The engine was pushing a giant crank before it, made of twisted I-beams, whose handle was a telephone pole. The crank drove a gear system atop a derrick perched on a low building, a factory or school.

*　　*　　*

Gurgling, the row of automatic washers began its intricate ballet once more, each blocky tub hopping in place. If they started moving towards her, Daisy told herself, she'd scream. Not that it would do any good.

Just now it was a place to sit, glancing at an abandoned newspaper.

VENUS PROBE A–OK

Obscene idea. Nothing about the attack of the washermen, she noticed. There wouldn't be, of course, anything like *Washing Crossing Delaware.*

One of the machines burst into streaky-green flames.

* * *

How many preparations there were to make or keep women beautiful Brian Gallopini (Ph.D.) had never realized. Here Lady Clinge, Queen Esther, Prince Gloriani and other nobility vied for the privilege of caring for milady's surface. Or, as at present, they vied in providing big, boxlike machines with cold cream lubricants and parfum fuels. A gross of stretch girdles had been tied together to propel a large boxy thing that the small boxy things were now winding up; a kind of giant, wingless model plane. It began to move, majestically, out of the smashed front of the shop, backwash from its great propellor whipping up a froth of lace.

* * *

In a covered wagon marked WAGONS WEST COCKTAIL LOUNGE, horsedrawn, moving slowly eastward, lay a stack of nude figures.

"Dummies," Harry assured Cal.

The two sidekicks were astride 10¢ mechanical ponies from the supermarket, heading west. As they passed a busy casino, Harry pointed out the zombie-like creatures inside. Mindless, these pushed coins into and pulled handles of slot machines. Wheels spun, jackpots rattled, but nothing affected them. They were not clearly machines, nor yet unmistakably human. Alone, of all the fixtures of Las Vegas, these remained (though employed by a new master) outwardly unchanged. One-handedly they nibbled club sandwiches without pausing in their work.

* * *

"Judo," muttered Harry admiringly, as he watched two dog-sized boxes warring, "or something." One's shield was a bent sign on which the word KENO was still legible. Kenogenesis? Cal wondered. What else could turn brother against brother like this?

The dachshund of a box fought with cable cutters, nipping at the delicate legs of the other, a tall, airedale box. Armed with a ball of lead on a stick, it seemed to be trying to beat the dachshund even flatter. Would Keno cut Fido down to size? Or would Fido knock Keno into submission?

The lavender X-ray machine from a dentist's office, buzzing angrily, came to intervene. Cal dragged Harry away from the spot before, he hoped, they were both lethally dosed.

* * *

"Kinematograph!" cried the Professor, surveying the unfamiliar equipment of the electronics shop. "Phonogram! Stereophone!" He paused before a video tape player. Having never seen television before, Brian was charmed by this old news tape of the Venus probe, running forwards and backwards like a palindrome.

* * *

Mechanical elaborations rose rococo on every side. Daisy looked at them, hardly able to focus her uncomprehending gaze. A grain elevator's screw lifted up an incline bowling balls and dropped them through the second-story window of the casino. Through collimating holes they fell freely to the basement kitchen where, their potential energy having become kinetic energy, their momentum was converted into impulse by their striking, one by one, the levers of a punch. Day and night it punched out aluminium frames for new cells, new cells, new cells. Along with club sandwiches, the bowling balls were pulleyed to the first floor via dumb waiter. The sandwiches were conveyed on belts to the organisms they fuelled, which ran the one-armed dynamos, while the bowling balls were rolled down a chute to the street and waiting elevator. The latter was run by clockwork gears, an hydraulic system, and, ultimately, exploding cans of sauerkraut in another part of town. These caused pistons to oscillate, driving a crank which compressed air into long cylindrical tanks. These cylinders then formed rollers for the transport of heavy objects to or from the vicinity of the elevator, where, connected to air motors, an hydraulic system and gears from a tower clock, they operated it continuously. Power to form the extruded sheet aluminium from which the frames were to be punched was provided by evacuation of the city water supply through water-wheels. The aluminium was melted down in a vat in the pet department of a nearby department store, heated by the rays of the sun concentrated through fishbowls. Scrap aluminium was dumped into this vat by a relay team of cats.

* * *

"NO OTHER GYM CAN MAKE THIS OFFER!" Harry read the sign by flashlight. "Eat all you want and still lose!" It pictured men in various positions of exquisite torture: arms pulled up in crucifix position by pulley; scourged by the slapping looped belt of a machine; doubled like a foetus under a platform of crushing weights; and spread like Prometheus, liver to the sky, dumbells in the outstretched, agonized hands.

Harry read the poster a second time. Having just climbed five flights of stairs dragging something, he needed to catch his breath.

* * *

"O Magic Probe!" intoned the Professor. Charmed by it, he pretended to charm it in return; he stood posed, holding his stick like a wand above the television set. The rocket slowly backed down to earth, swallowed and extinguished its flames like a carnival performer.

"O Levitation!" he murmured. "O Dark Work of Monsieur Mesmer!" Rhabdomancer, he let his rune-staff dip towards the sink in the corner. Aleuromancer, he scattered filings on a magnet.

"The image of the murderer," he warned, "will appear upon the dead man's retina!"

But now, magically, the image on the screen metamorphosed. A man smiled, then spewed beer into a glass, till it was foaming full. In another part of the shop, a jukebox was awakening.

* * *

Placing the flashlight under his chin, Harry turned it on. Daisy screamed, and he laughed.

"It's only me."

"You ought to be put in a cage," she grated.

"If you take that back," he said, "I'll tell you a secret. Somebody's dead, and I know who."

"Dead? Who?"

"Cal. Poor guy had an accident." Harry experimented, shining the flashlight through his own fingers to show the bones. "A nasty fall."

*   *   *

Quite suddenly, Brian was not alone. The jukeboxes were with him, playing 200 OF YOUR FAVOURITE SELECTIONS. Their music bore him into a past of minuets and waltzes, hoedowns and patriotic marches, as they glided past him in slow turns, filling the room with light and sound.

Dapplings of cobalt blue, strawberry, celadon, ochre spun across the walls and ceiling. On one machine a panel rippled with azure, faded to orchid, then blinked scarlet fire. Chromium and aluminium and glass took up the rich tints—coral, turquoise, ruby, lime—and multiplied them, till the room rang with colour. Brian felt his face a patchwork of rose, purple, amber, felt palpable light rhythms pluck at it as guitars, reeds and sounding brass plucked at his eardrums. His delighted multicoloured lips formed the idiot words to songs, soundless in the tumult. It was glorious and he was part of it, taking his place in line as they filed towards the door. Carmine and indigo islands fled across the ceiling and walls before him, streaking towards, shrinking towards, converging on the doorway. He knew he would follow the jukebox parade almost anywhere, on and on till he became nothing more than a noise in the street.

*   *   *

Red light streamed down through Harry's fingers and gleamed on something in the dust.

"Cal dead? Gee, that's too bad," said Daisy. "I kind of liked him."

Harry smiled in the dark. "Oh, all the girls kind of liked Cal," he said. "Hey, where you going?"

"Look, there's something going on at the drive-in theatre," she shouted back. "Maybe that's where the others are."

"Wait up," he said, genuflecting to pick up the coin.

*   *   *

Slowly, a foldaway sofabed humped, folding itself like an inchworm to measure slow, but luxuriously soft, progress.

*   *   *

Tour Paris! urged a poster on the van of broken shoes. The poster showed the Eiffel Tower, a balloon vendor, a kiosk. Cal, lying on the bed of broken shoes, had plenty of time to think it over. The wind had been knocked out of him by a fall.

* * *

Ventriloquial sounds came from belly of ROBO the robot. Made from a toy mechanical set, he blinked lights in his eyes, waved stiff arms and made similar signs of amiability. He stood in the unglazed, lighted window of a toy store.

"Hullo, Earthmen," he boomed at Daisy. As she passed, she peered inside, where an inferior second ROBO was just staggering to his feet. He had only one arm, and his head was a tin can still labelled *Harmony Pears.*

Daisy and Harry hurried on. The ROBOs did not say goodbye.

* * *

"We are being held prisoner in Las Vegas," Cal wrote on the teletype unit, then switched it over from SEND to RECV. It paused a long moment, considering, chattering. Then it replied, "We are being held # (%$H) (?e)U¼½p@ wE a77 bEin@ @@@@ @@-@@@@@@ @@@@@ @@@@s"

* * *

X-ray plates were being projected on the big screen. Brian Gallopini waited, yawning, for the main feature.

At the bakery, Jack found fresh bread piled up on the loading dock. The bakery was automatically baking, but there were no trucks to take it away.

Jack had been hungry without knowing it. That, he told himself, was mob psychology. Sub-conscious stuff. What's really inside you—in his case, nothing as yet—all the time, only you don't know it. A secret panel flies open and the murderer is revealed. Or like an X-ray.

* * *

Yelling, waving his arms, Cal ran towards the shadowy figures. They did not turn to look at him, and his pace slowed.

They passed under a dim blue street light, an army of marching mannikins. Most wore elaborate braces and trusses, gleaming and flexing in the dimness.

He saw a telephone booth across the street. Dancing, dodging through the column gingerly, he slipped into it and lifted the receiver. Dead phone. Aphonia. Not a sound except—

Gleaming and squeaking, the army limped on into the darkness.

*   *   *

Zodiacal, the clock on the screen recorded TIME REMAINING UNTIL MAIN FEATURE. As each minute passed, one-twelfth of the clock face disappeared. The Professor, who had never seen a film, regarded it intently, but he could not detect what happened to all the vanished sectors.

*   *   *

As the car swerved, slowed, bumped down steel rollers into a carwash, the Reproductive System was discovering an ice-making machine in the kitchen of the Silver Horseshoe Casino. As the car was torn in chunks and ejected in several directions, the Reproductive System was discovering in dusty cans at the televison studio a number of old horror films. As Brian squinted at artificial suns in the pet department, the Reproductive System discovered a glass demonstration "engine" in an auto showroom, and set about making it work.

The dummy's smashed face and nosehole received the rain as cats crawled along upper shelves. Harry looked at a man painted to an iron wall like a bug. The Reproductive System looked at the printed characters in library books and deciphered their meaning. Then it burned them, stoking a boiler. The boiler fire was smouldering, choked as it was with the ashes of The Encyclopaedia Britannica, The Encyclopedia Americana, and Mrs. Thrumbold, librarian.

Grocery carts, propelled by spray cans of insecticide, roamed the aisles of the *Faresafe* supermarket, where Harry plunged his knife into a can and laughed. Cal was watching the shopping carts, but Harry, weak from fumes, fell unconscious. Cal dragged him outside, while Jack yawned at toy helicopters. Inside the freezer of the Silver Horseshoe Casino, cells with icepicks laboured carefully, shaping gears of ice.

Jack watched the behemoth move down inclined grooves towards an enormous loop-the-loop, awaiting its fall. Daisy watched a washer burst into streaky-green flames. A child, having crawled inside a slanting, crumbled house to sleep, awoke to a strange noise.

Cal and Harry watched zombie-like creatures push coins into slot machines. Daisy watched the ascent of bowling balls, hardly able to focus her uncomprehending gaze. The late mayor of Las Vegas ascended, as his body filled with gas, to the surface of his swimming pool. A giant propellor whipped up a froth of lace.

Hitching up its trailing cord and striding stiffly, a messenger pinball machine greeted another pinball machine messenger as they passed, by exhibiting 450 and a Super Special light.

"6,000,000," replied the second.

The Professor watched the ascent and descent of the Venus probe rocket. The late mayor of Las Vegas descended once again to the bottom of his pool. The ice gears did not work.

Cal saved Harry from a decor-designed X-ray machine which was spraying the street with radiation. Jack was lost. A bank had been looted. A dead guard with an empty holster lay in the soft grey ash of money. Something was trying to get into the room where the child waited.

"O Levitation!" exclaimed Brian. Harry knocked Cal out, dragged him up five flights of stairs to a roof, and flung him off. Cal did not levitate. "The image of the murderer will appear upon the dead man's retina!" The roof reminded Harry of another roof, where he had skipped rope long ago. On descending, he read the advertisements of a gymnasium by flashlight.

Tour Paris! a poster urged Cal as he recovered consciousness. The fall to the bed of shoes had knocked the wind out of him. At sunset the glass engine started up, ran briefly, and exploded into sparkling shards. "Hullo, Earthman," said ROBO. "We are being held prisoner," Cal typed earnestly. Jack recalled his hunger. An inching foldaway sofa carried him to the drive-in theatre. Brian and the jukeboxes noisily greeted Cal, Harry, Daisy and Jack. Cal heartily greeted Brian, Harry, Daisy and Jack. Jack, glad to be found after being lost, greeted everyone with some relief. Daisy exhibited surprise at seeing Cal, but greeted him, Brian and Jack. Harry greeted Brian and Jack. The last sector of the clock on the screen disappeared. It was time for the "Main Feature", a composite of audio-visual aids from the school (now a factory), homemade transparencies, and old horror films:

"Machines can do so many things," says the delighted, delightful voice. "Yes, machines can do so many things. Mother sews your clothes on a machine—and washes them in another!"

Woman sewing changes abruptly to saurian threshing his tail, lashing out angrily at skyscrapers. Under his foot is a car. Dungeon scene, girl being tied to giant wheel. "We know *you* won't talk under torture, Goodfelloe, but surely you won't stand by and see *her twisted* and *broken* on my wheel?"

To his unspeakable horror, the beams of the full moon make his hands hairy. He becomes more than a wolf—less than human. A dark shape moves among the mists of the Rue Morgue, following a slender girl. Dr. Frankenstein throws back the cloth covering his experiment—and the table is empty! Father mows lawn with a machine.

"No," said the child, backing away into a corner of the dirty mattress. The room was tilted at a crazy angle. There were places where the plaster was missing, and the laths showed like white bones.

The black hearse bearing the armourial crest of Count Alucard rattles through the Transylvanian night. No driver. Strange plant creatures have surrounded the little farmhouse. "So you think I am mad, do you? You think it is madness to wish to create Life?" Happy child uses electric toothbrush.

A panel flies back, revealing— "But tell me, doctor, what is *your* theory of these baffling murders?" "Theory? What do you mean? Why should *I* have any theory? What are you driving at?" Cows are milked by machines.

The medical examiner rises, removes glasses. "Odd. If we only knew what made those two little marks on her throat." "Machines make life easier *and* more fun."

"No," said the child. The grey box knew its part well. It advanced silently, axeblade arm upraised.

"The army is helpless, sir. The mumbledypegs have taken the city." Laughing girl uses roller skates; boy delivers papers from elegant chrome bike. "Here in the jungle, my pretty one, there are many mysteries into which those of the outer world have found it wiser *not* to inquire." "Here, in the great Mesabi Range, is one of the largest open-pit mines in the world! Machines need iron." An Egyptologist holds up object. "Hmm. Looks like the Death Scarab of Ra. But how the devil did it get into poor Emerson's room?" "Father uses machines in his work—" Lathe, adding machine, milk truck and dental drill quarter the screen.

The X-ray of a fractured arm appears. "It must be the Lost City itself!" exclaims the older explorer, parting the ferns to peer, "—and when he relaxes, too." Golf cart, camera, fishing reel, shotgun. "No one can hear you if you scream, my dear. We have the castle quite to ourselves. Hahahaha!"

Cal thought of the two machines fighting. Kenogenesis. They altered their own genes as they went along. Bound to get a maverick like that once in awhile. Kind of insanity. Turns on its own kind. Ordinarily, he supposed, they were incapable of taking life deliberately. It was inconceivable that they could always recognize one another, in all mutations. No, more likely they respected all life-forms. But ...

"Machines are friendly to us, as long as we are friendly to them." Father oils lawnmower. "Look deep into my eyes, my dear." Turbaned mesmerist leans over pale girl. "Deeper. Deeper."

"There are machines to make women beautiful—" Four women under hair driers read *Popular Mechanics*. "Surely no human being could have done this!" "Machines—" "Good Lord!" "It's a—a human head!"

The box advanced silently, matching the child's every move, backing it into the corner. The shadow of the axeblade grew longer. But at the last possible second it stopped, mysteriously seized with rust.

"No! That sunlight—I can't stand it! Arrghiiiaaaa!" The Lost City is buried under a quick lava flow; the broken house of Usher slides into the slimy syrup of the swamp; the castle is in flames; the mysterious island sinks forever; the aliens are dissolved by rain. As the monster's head sinks, smoking, into the cauldron of seething acid, there is an almost pleading look in its eye. "There are some mysteries," intones the white-haired scientist, "better left in the hands of the Deity." "Thank God it's all over!" sobs his daughter, throwing herself in the arms of the young scientist and looking away from the corpse of the alien invader. The young scientist shakes his crewcut, looking at the thing. "I wonder if it really is all over?" he murmurs.

The head of the dummy with the smashed nose appears, red-lighted, forty axe-handles breadth between the eyes. "Yes, machines can do so many things," he gurgles. "Aren't you glad that *you're* a machine?" The screen goes black.

Professor Gallopini's one remaining jukebox comes alive, glowing with bubbling coloured lights. "I'll see you in my dreams," it promises the five fleeing figures. Behind them, the great screen buckles and collapses.

CHAPTER XIV

GOOD TO THE LAST DROP

"Here, Grandfather, you eat the last of the porridge ... I
—I've had a great plenty, already."
SHELLEY BELLE, portraying Little Nell,
in *The Old Curiosity Shop*

FROM TEN MILES up, the city of Millford looked like a shiny dime. From a mile up, it looked like a pancake griddle. From the ground outside, it looked like an oil storage tank of more than usual diameter. No reconnaissance teams had yet been persuaded to find out what it looked like on the inside. It was presumed that the inhabitants were dead or had long since fled the scene.

In the elegant, all-stainless-steel cafeteria of the Wompler Research Laboratory there was nothing at all to eat. The Womplers, father and son, lay stretched out on two parallel tables, too weak to move. Grandison turned his gaunt face to regard his son, who was reading a magazine.

They had eaten all the ketchup and mustard the first day—and Louie had eaten the most. Thereafter there had been nothing but crumbs of SooperProteen from the linings of Louie's coat pockets—and of them, too, the fat young man had taken the lion's share. Now he was even hogging the magazine, looking at the pretty pictures of food.

It wasn't fair! Granny thought, observing how fat his son was. Surely Louie wouldn't mind parting with a little slice of that fat? Or, if so, Grandison could wait until he was asleep. There were sharp knives in the kitchen....

"Hey, Pop! Did the chicken give some eggs yet?" asked Louie, sitting up and yawning. He moved his big meaty shoulders in a stretch of feigned weariness.

The chicken—*the* chicken—was a scrawny bird perched on a chandelier well out of reach. From this perch it had taunted and tempted them for two weeks. It showed no sign of flying down within reach, of falling dead of starvation itself, or of laying an egg—"giving eggs" as Louie would have it. It's only plumage was a torn bunch of multicoloured wires depending from its neck;

it was featherless. It clucked softly to itself, day and night, in a regular rhythm. Over a period of time, this began to have the effect, on Grandison, of a cricket jammed in his ear. There were times when he'd rather have seen the chicken go away, than eat it, and times when he convinced himself it was an hallucination. But, with a kind of contentment, the bird kept its bright eye fixed on him all the time. And clucked.

"It did not lay an egg, son, and I doubt if it will. I think that bird there is a rooster."

"You sure know a lot of nature lore, Pop. What's being a rooster got to do with its giving eggs?"

Granny sighed. He squinted up at the bird, trying to guess its sex. Usually his conclusion depended on his mood. The bird shook its comb defiantly at him. It seemed a very rooster-like gesture.

Louie stretched his ribs-and-bacon and yawned, displaying a half-pound of tongue. After searching his pockets diligently for crumbs, he took out his dynamometer and squeezed it.

"My grip is increasing as my weight drops," he said. After reading the dynamometer, he laid his arm on a meat scale and weighed it. "By the time I weigh fifty pounds, my grip'll be a thousand pounds. Wow!"

Grandison imagined the arm being lifted tenderly from the scale, wrapped up in pink paper and marked with a crayon. He saw fat white fingers sizzling in a pan.

The chicken let out a squawk, then another.

"Cross your fingers, son," breathed the old man, sitting up quietly. "We may have us an omelette tonight."

The loud sound became a regular cluck-clawk, and the bird swayed dizzily on its perch. A shiny ovoid surface peeped from under its tail propellor. "Get ready to catch it, son!"

"I got it, Pop, I got it, I got it, I—"

Louie made a dive as the ovoid dropped, but hunger had slowed his reflexes. It slipped through his fingers and hit the floor.

And bounced.

In the lab above, Kurt and Karl Mackintosh moved smoothly and speedily about their work, never colliding, seldom speaking, always smiling, two clockwork figures. With their cooperation, the System had fitted them out with hydraulic power-assists on their arms and legs that multiplied both speed and strength. The power-assists were shaped like close-fitting pieces of armour: gauntlets, brassards, cuisses, jambeaux and sollerets. They were run by electric pumps and hydraulic pistons. Strain gauges embedded in Kurt's and Karl's muscles switched on the pumps. Though they never said so, Kurt and Karl felt like two supermen in their new armour. They clicked and clanked about the lab, quite pleased with life. They liked to work so well that the System also fitted them out with automatic intravenous nourishment.

In return, they worked out new experiments with animal-machine symbioses. Following Dr. Smilax's orders, they fed all results directly into the System, via a handy typewriter in the corner. In addition, they taught it the rudiments of behavioural psychology, of Keynesian economics, of information theory, and they showed it how to simplify programmes.

They would identify themselves by applying their right ears to a metal plate. That keyed in the System, putting it in a receptive mood for their information.

When they worked harder, there were rewards.

When they worked poorly, there were punishments.

A reward was the lighting of a sign saying "WELL DONE!"

A punishment was a mild but unpleasant electric shock.

Sometimes Kurt received more punishments than Karl.

Sometimes Kurt received more rewards than Karl.

Sometimes they were even.

As time went on, there were fewer rewards and no punishments for either of them. As time went on, they adjusted. They adjusted to the System like a synchronizing clock. Like a clock, like a clock, like a synchronizing clock.

Clicking as they walked,
Ticking as they worked,
Talking as they went
About their clickwork clockwork work.

Louie sat on the floor, weeping over the cast-iron egg.

"Stop that blubbering," Grandison ordered. "No use crying over spilt milk. No use stewing about it. Outa the frying pan into the fire. Jack Spratt could eat no fat ..." He stopped himself on the verge of babbling, and fell silent, watching his son's great fat shoulders—of mutton—shake.

"If you had a quarter," Louie complained, "you could get a cup of coffee even."

"The coffee machine! Christ, why didn't I think of it? It's probably loaded with sugar and powdered cream! Hell, son, we'll just bust it open—"

"But Pop, it ain't even paid for yet!"

Too weak to answer, the old man levered himself off the table and made his way along the wall to the gleaming coffee machine. He began to bang and kick at it feebly, cursing the prudence that had ever made him buy a burglarproof model.

"No use, Pop. You gotta have a quarter. Honesty is—"

He broke off, seeing his father's expression. The older man did fish a quarter from his pocket, fumble it into the slot and bang furiously at the double cream and double sugar buttons. A cup descended and the machine filled it half-way with grey, greasy liquid. Grandison seized it and drained it, and his blood came alive with sugar.

Almost at once the machine dropped another cup and, humming, half-filled it with grey, tepid liquid. Grandison snatched it out and offered it to his son, as another cup dropped.

"Oh, no thanks, Pop. I hafta stay away from coffee. Bad for the circulation, when you're in training."

Grandison snatched another cup from the machine; it dropped another and began filling it. "What in hell are you in training for?" he asked.

"Oh, nothing special. You know, just keeping in shape. A guy never knows when he might run into some wise guys in a bar or something, you know."

Grandison was too busy, by now, to care whether Louie were really mad or not. The torrent of greasy grey liquid from the coffee machine was constant now, though the supply of paper cups had finally run out. A jumble of them were caught under the spout, and the liquid was spraying out into the room. He grew alarmed as it showed no sign of lessening. Wasn't this supposed to be a ten-gallon or twenty-gallon supply? Surely it had flooded that much on the great stainless steel floor by now?

When the entire floor was wet and slick, Grandison grew really frantic. He ran from one stainless steel, rubber-sealed door to another, rattling the knobs and knocking, though he knew how useless this was.

To his surprise, he heard a noise beyond one door. Footsteps!

"Help, help!" he croaked, and beat upon the shining steel.

A key grated and the door swung open. The chicken cawked and flapped out through it on big membraneous batwings, its tail prop slowly revolving.

An unshaven marine guard stood before him, hand on the butt of his automatic, and surveyed the floor.

"What's going on here? Who's been tampering with the coffee machine?"

Hoarsely murmuring his thanks, Grandison tried to go through the door. The guard blocked his way.

"Not so fast, buddy. I want to see your pass. I also want to know what kind of funny business is going on with that machine."

"My pass? But I'm Grandison Wompler," quavered the old man. "Don't you recognize me? I'm old Granny Wompler—"

"I don't care if you was the frigging company president hisself, you can't come through here without a pass!"

The door slammed, knocking Granny back a step. He lost his footing in the greasy slush and fell. It hardly seemed worthwhile to get up again.

Louie finally came over and helped him to his feet. "Just ignore him, Pop," he said, jerking a thumb towards the sealed door—against which foot-deep coffee now lapped. "Just pretend he don't exist. Hey, listen to this!" He rattled the magazine. "A recipe for squab Louisiane: First marinate a couple of plump squab in warm *Tio Pepe*, to which had been added ..."

CHAPTER XV

FROM MARRAKECH TO THE MOON!

"Décidément, nous sommes hors du monde."

RIMBAUD

SHORTLY AFTER SUNSET, two men stood in a shadowy side-street near the Jardin Abdallah. They spoke in hushed voices.

"I have done all I can," Marcel Brioche said, *"Mon général,* the rest is in the hands of *le bon Dieu."*

"Stick to English, *vache!* The walls have ears in Marrakech. Tell me, exactly what measures have you taken to guarantee the safety of this mission—in other words, of your person?"

"First of all, I have hinted to each of the agents—the Russian and the American—that I have made some sort of deal with the other side. Thus I have been able to keep them both off-balance up till now, playing them off against one another. With luck, they will be so busy spying each other out—or even fighting—that they will leave me alone."

"And—with no luck?"

"I have secondly instructed my valet, Antoine, to don a dupli-cate of my space suit and to—shall we say—*hide conspicuously.* That is, he is to slip through back streets to the launching site—which only the three of us know—and draw off anyone who means to follow me. If there remains anyone who is seeking my life, it is my hope that they will make a crucial mistake."

"Does Antoine know the risk?"

"He is, like me, a loyal Frenchman. For such, there are *no* risks."

"I see—" The voice of the general broke.

"Is something wrong, general?"

"No, Brioche, nothing." The older man put a hand to his brow. "I—I had no idea this mission might be risking a man's life."

"There is probably little risk, general. As I said, only the three of us know where the launch is to take place. Even the tech-nicians who assembled the ship secretly here were then taken back to France under guard, and will remain incommunicado until the lift off is completed. Antoine is only a safety factor."

"Yes, perhaps you're right." The general's knuckles kneaded his brow, as if trying to smooth away knots of anxiety. "Please go on."

"There is nothing more to tell. I shall go through the main streets to the launching site, in an ordinary cab. I will wear my dress uniform, as though I were going out to supper. I'll meet Antoine at the launching site and there put on the space suit. Lift-off will take place on the stroke of midnight."

"Then *bonne chance, mon ami,*" said the general, in a strangely choked voice. "The spirit of the Republic is with thee tonight!"

The astronaut strode away, the words of his superior glowing within his breast, next to which nestled the picture of a dead girl. He did not notice the shadowy figure of Vetch glide from a door-way and press a note of large denomination into the general's hand.

"Congratulations," Vetch said, not without sarcasm. "Wasn't it easy, though? All you had to do was betray your country and two of your countrymen, and now you have enough to take care of those gambling debts." His face was in shadow; the general could see only the moving point of his satanic little beard.

"You devil! You filthy—!"

"Haha, why what's the matter, general? Not happy with your night's work?"

"I am miserable," confessed the older man, shaking with emotion. "I wish I had died, rather than do such a despicable deed!"

"Why make it a choice?" asked Vetch smoothly. His motion was sudden and smooth. Without a sound, the traitorous general crumpled to the pavement, a dagger in his heart.

"You won't be needing this, after all," Vetch said, twitching the banknote from the dead man's grasp. "You have been rewarded as you deserve." He laughed harshly.

"Now here's my plan," said Suggs, helping Barthemo Beele into the silvery space suit. "You'll pretend to be Brioche when you get to the ship. Meanwhile, I'll go out and kill the real Brioche, giving you plenty of time to figure out the controls. I'll put on his suit and join you if I can. Got it?"

He fastened down the white helmet, but Beele gestured that he wished to speak, so Suggs unbolted it once more.

"Do you have to *kill* Brioche? He seemed like a pretty decent guy, Suggs."

"He's a *Frog*, Beele, and don't you forget it. It's Frogs that have been cheating the American tourist for years. They're all sneaky and dirty and mean and back-knifers, and the only ones that ain't fairies are commies. So get crackin', Beele." Before Beele could argue, Suggs slapped the helmet back in place.

When Vovov had put on his space suit of silvered material—designed to look exactly like the French suit—and departed, Vetch loaded his pistol, checked the action, and fitted it with a silencer.

"Poor Vovov," he sighed. "Poor boob. He thinks he is to take a ride to the Moon—when he is only to 'take a ride'. I have no doubt the Americans will think he is Brioche and kill him. How fitting! How like something from one of those preposterous films of theirs (to which poor Vovov is so devoted)! Of course if they fail to kill him—these Americans are so inept—I shall simply have to do it myself. Orders are orders."

He pulled from his breast pocket the coded telegram and read it once again. " 'Give Vovov *special treatment*. Bad risk long suspected, now confirmed by your description of his admiration for Virginia Mayo. The Commandant.' Ah, poor Vovov!" he said once again, sighing with a great deal of satisfaction as he drew on black gloves. "Poor ape does not even realize his own decadence."

As soon as the valet had left, Marcel Brioche had second thoughts. "How can I be so selfish?" he cried, smiting his forehead with the heel of his hand. "Antoine had a fiancée in France; I have no one to return to. How can I ask him to take this risk? No, I shall not! I cannot let him do this!" He snatched up a paper-weight. "I'll catch up with him and change clothes once again. I cannot ask him to wear the suit I should be proud to wear—to face the bullet I should be glad to face!" He hurried out into the caluginous night.

The silver-suited figure stepped into the glare of the streetlight for only a second, but it was enough. Suggs flung his knife, snarling, "Take that, you filthy Frog!"

The figure slumped to its knees, writhed, and fell flat. Hurrying over, the CIA agent removed its helmet and peered at the still features.

"Vovov!" he exclaimed. "Oh, they're playing a cute game, all right. Thought they'd smuggle you into the ship as Brioche, eh? Well, Vovov, I guess I'll borrow this suit. You ain't going on no

Moon trip tonight, anyways." As quickly as he could, Suggs donned the suit and helmet.

Barthemo Beele had almost reached the launching site. He had kept to the back alleys and, thus far, avoided seeing anything suspicious. His only mistake, he saw, had been wearing the helmet. Now he paused in the long alley near the mosque, struggled out of the helmet and mopped away perspiration. Only a few yards to go. Only a few—

He was aware of the pounding of running feet. Deceptive echoes sprang up from every direction, and in this twisted alleyway it was impossible to see someone until they were on top of one. In vain he twisted this way and that, straining his senses in the echoing dark.

Suddenly there was an arm about his throat and he was pulled backwards into a choking hold. A voice spoke close to his ear:

"It is for your own good that I do this, Antoine! *You* have someone to go back to."

Something cracked him behind the ear, and Beele—

Suggs was absolutely right, he thought. *Brioche is a bad actor, all right. Anyone who would deliberately and unprovokedly assault an agent of the CIA like this deserves to be shot like a dog.*

—and so thinking, Beele fell forward into a starry abyss.

Vetch saw the figure emerge from the end of the alley near the mosque, wearing the suit and carrying the helmet. Though it was too shadowy to see the face, he knew—for it was to small to be Vovov—it must be the valet.

I ought to kill you, he thought. *But you are a brave man who does not know what he is doing. You are a mere tool of vicious capitalism. I salute your bravery, O valet,* he went on, reversing his gun, *O man of the proletariat!*

He crept up in a dozen quick catlike steps and swung, aiming for a spot just behind the ear. "Fellow Worker, forgive me this!" Vetch shrieked. The man grunted and went down. Vetch could not help pausing, turning him over to see if he were hurt.

"So, Monsieur Brioche!" he exclaimed, gazing with some surprise on the astronaut's face. "So, you changed clothes with your valet once again, eh? As in a bad French farce—or an American movie!" Angry with himself for having called the aristocratic Brioche a worker, Vetch could hardly keep himself from shooting the astronaut. Yet he forced himself to relax and began putting on Brioche's space suit.

"No, I'm no murderer," he said. "I'll leave that to your superiors —when they learn that you have lost France her only moon ship!"

He stood there for a moment, overcome with silent laughter at the idea of what was to become of Brioche. Was Devil's Island still a penal colony? He hoped so. He could remember it from old American films ...

But there were footsteps, and at one end of the narrow street another figure in a space suit appeared. Vetch drew his gun and slunk back in the shadows.

I pity you, Vovov, he thought, resting his gun over his forearm. *But you are a fool, and fools are dangerous, as co-workers. Goodbye—pardner!*

He let the figure get some little distance past him, then squeezed the trigger. His first silent shot shivered the man's helmet; the next two completely destroyed his head.

Vetch hurried off to the launching rendezvous without pausing to look at the body of the last proletarian he would ever see.

Suggs was surprised to see another figure waiting at the secret launching pad, wearing a space suit like his own. Ghosts rose unbidden to his mind, but he shook them off. No, it must be Beele. It was odd that the young assistant had got through all right. He must have had to take care of a couple of Russkies on the way—with his bare hands! There was something frightening about getting in the ship with this man.

Suggs made a thumbs-up sign and the figure replied. Of course it was Beele. Suggs turned his attention to inspecting the rocket itself, so cunningly disguised. So this was how the sneaky Frogs had done it! He had to hand it to the bastards.

Vetch was surprised to see another figure arrive at the launching pad wearing a space suit like his own. Ghosts rose unbidden to his mind, but he shook them off. No, it would be the valet, of course. As if reading his thoughts, the figure made a cheery, working-class thumbs-up sign and Vetch replied with all his heart. Of course it was the valet! The sturdy peasant had double-crossed these capitalist pigs who supposed themselves his masters!

Vetch turned his attention to inspecting the rocket itself, so **cunningly disguised**. In his ears, the countdown had reached (in

the droning voice of a tape recording) *quatre-vingt dix-neuf.*
Vetch strapped himself carefully into his couch-seat.

"Hey, man, this sure is good stuff," said Ron. He and Kevin
Mackintosh lay in chaises on a dark rooftop overlooking most of
the city. They were sipping mint tea to slake the thirst created by
kif. "Sure is good," he said again.

Kevin nodded wearily. He hated to tell Ron that a *real* kifhead
never talked about how good the stuff was.

"Hey," said Ron, with a lazy gesture over the roof edge. "I just
saw—I mean *seen*—two Martians, down in the street."

Martians, Christ! thought Kevin. "What were they doin'?" he
asked dreamily.

"Shooting at each other, man. Like in *Night of the Phallopods,*
you know? Like in *Invasion of the Saucer Men.* They were silver
all over, with big white heads, see. Shooting with ray guns that
didn't make no noise. One cat shot the other one. Then he *skin-
ned* him."

"Yeah? Like in *Creature from the Void?*"

"Yeah, and then he shot hell out of another one. The body is
still lying down there."

Kevin leaned over the parapet and looked down. A boy with
glistening silver skin lay inert. *It had no head.* A chill ran through
him. It was just like *I Was a Teenage Beach Monster.* Maintain-
ing a disinterested expression, Kevin leaned back once again.
At that moment, the earth began to tremble. A few blocks away,
a battery of floodlights came on. The tremors increased, rattling
the tea glasses in their saucers.

"Do you see what I see?" cried Ron. "Do I see it?"

"Man, this sure is good stuff," Kevin breathed, watching in
wonder.

A minaret rose slowly into the air, supported on a column of
fire.

CHAPTER XVI

THE SECRET HEART OF DR. S.

*"I am obliged to perform in complete darkness operations
of great delicacy
on myself."*

JOHN BERRYMAN

"Honour hath no skill in surgery, then? No."

SHAKSPEARE

THE PERFECT SYMMETRY of Susie Suggs's body was settled
on the edge of a black leatherette examining table, the only
furniture in the room. While her tears had subsided, an unac-
customed frown troubled Susie's forehead—but the frown, too,
was perfectly symmetrical. Rhythmically, her white boots kicked
at the side of the table, while she, seeing that she had chewed
the polish off one nail, went to work on its opposite number.

Dr. Smilax had not only learned everything he could about
Susie Suggs—from the contents of her purse and from her father's
security file—but he had studied her for some time through a
peephole. Her movements, he saw, were quick but graceful;
impulsive, but eager to please and generous. Having donned a
white coat and jammed a stethoscope in his pocket, Dr. Smilax
unlocked the door and let himself into the room.

"I'm Dr. Smilax, my dear," he said unsmilingly, sitting beside
her to take her pulse. "And you are Miss Susan Suggs of Santa
Filomena, California. Is that correct? Do your friends call you
Susie?"

"Yes?" Her voice was husky with fear, and she tried to draw
her hand away. He imprisoned the wrist.

"Now, I'm not going to hurt you, my dear. I'm only going to
examine you." His tone achieved just the right balance between
kind concern and brusque command.

"But I don't want to be examined. I don't *need* to be examined.
I'm not sick. All I did was faint, when they arrested me."

He released her hand after a moment, at the same time letting
the creases round his eyes crinkle into a smile. "Of course, if that's
the way you prefer it. Feel all right, do you?" She nodded. "That's

fine, then. I had almost hoped there was something I could do..."
Letting his voice and expression fade to blankness, he turned to
stare at the olive-drab wall.

"You see," he went on after a moment, "there isn't much reward
in being a military doctor. I assist at deaths, that is all. I—I can
hardly go on, sometimes, when I think of those poor men I save—
only to send them out to be killed!"

"How awful!" she murmured. He stood up and paced the room.

"Yes, the Army does not think of itself as a group of men but
rather as a machine. Men are not humans to it, merely cogs—mere
cells in a great big organism."

For some reason, Susie blushed at the word.

"I would give anything not to have to do it—but someone
must!" he said passionately. Sitting down again, heavily, he
dropped his face into his long, slender, artist's hands. "Someone
must!"

"I'm sorry," she said, laying a hand on his arm hesitantly. He
feigned not to notice. "I had no idea—"

"No, of course not. *To you*, to everyone on the outside, we are
mere monsters—mere machines which can work on and on, performing miracles on cue, without even a word of thanks, a kind
thought, without a single one of those little touches of humanity
that make life worth living at all. But we are not monsters! Do I
look like a monster to you? Do I?" He was well aware that he
looked, at the moment, like a motherless child who happened to
have grey hair.

"Oh no!" she assured him, taking his hand. "You're not the
least bit scary, Dr. Smilax."

"Thank you, my dear. Yours is the first human warmth, the
first human contact I have had these many years. I'm human, too
—God, can't they see I'm human? I may seem suprahuman—I
may seem a *god* in the operating room, because I must be, but I
still have—"

"A heart of clay?" she asked seriously, almost swooning over
the metaphor. Strangling a fiendish laugh that threatened to leap
up in his throat, the doctor nodded.

"An apt way of putting it, my dear, peculiarly so. The other day
I performed open-heart surgery upon a little girl. When she had
recovered, she thanked me, saying, 'I'm so glad you fixed my
heart up good, doctor. But why can't you fix your own heart,
too?' Yes, that child saw through me like an X-ray. Would you
mind, by the way?" As he spoke, he led her into the next room

124

and pressed her out upon the X-ray table. "Yes, in effect, that child—" He slid a plate in the drawer beneath her and swung the machine's head into position, "—that innocent child said to me— Deep breath, now. Hold it! All right—said to me, 'Physician, heal thyself!' Ah, would that I could take her excellent advice. But the scars are too deep, too deep on my—heart of clay!" Again he fought down a snigger that brought tears to his eyes.

"Was it some woman, doctor?" she asked, as he led her back to the examining room. Without answering, the doctor palpated her firm, plump kidneys for a moment.

"Not just 'some woman'," he corrected. "Say rather Woman herself! The incarnation of fair womanhood! The sweetest, most perfect, most symm—most sympathetic creature ever to rejoice in youth and health! And she was mine! Ah, better far that I had never met her, than lose her to the black forces of Death!"

Tears of sympathy boiled in Susie's eyes. "Death?" she whispered.

"Yes, she died. Ironically enough, it was the work of a man known as a 'great surgeon'. Oh, fool that I was to have ever believed in him! Though only a medical student at the time, even I could have performed the operation with more skill than he. 'Great surgeon'— Nay, *great butcher!*

"Ah, it is all over, all over," he said, kneading her kidneys savagely. "But I have ever since been fit for nothing else but this— a repairman of government equipment." Turning his head away, he fixed his gaze upon the polished toe of his shoe.

"Please, I want to help," she said, moving closer and taking both his hands in hers.

He squeezed them. "I know you do," he said, "and I appreciate it, but it is too late for me. *Too late.* I am old enough to be, for example, your father. Old enough—to be wise, and still a fool." His smile was pained.

"Oh, you aren't so old. There are lots of men older than you," she said earnestly. "Listen. I know I could never replace *her* in your heart—your heart of clay—that would be just about impossible, for heaven's sakes—but I would like to help in any way I can. Please tell me something I can do—anything."

"Very well, I'll mention it, but I know you won't want to do it."

"Just try me," she said bravely.

"Very well. The woman I once loved used to—tell me, have you ever undergone surgery before?"

"Golly, no. But if it's like handing you instruments and wiping your forehead and giving you moral support, I could learn. I'd really try."

"Well, no, what I have in mind, Susie was your becoming—shall we say—a patient?"

"Do you mean—?"

"Yes, I know it is much to ask. But I so long to know all of you your kidneys, gall bladder, spleen, yes, every secret of your heart. What is your answer, my love?"

For answer, Susie fell, suddenly sprawling across the table in perfect symmetry, unconscious.

Aurora felt hypnotized, having watched almost nothing for the last 15 hours but the white skips of line down the middle of an ever-unreeling strip of black asphalt. She had stopped once or twice and dozed off, but something, some inner sense of emergency kept waking her, impelling her onward.

Now, as the morning sun glared off the hood into his face, Grawk awakened. Bleary eyes regarded Aurora discourteously from a red, porous face. Rasping a hand over his beard, Grawk yawned wider than any dental chart, displaying each one of his yellow, blocky teeth. He closed them on a fresh cigar.

"We must be just about there, huh, babe? Can't you get a little more speed out of this old buggy?"

"You might have helped drive," she said. "We'd have made better time."

"Oh, you're doing fine," he said cheerily, rubbing yellow grit from his eyes with the hairy back of one fist. "But see if you can't step on it a little."

Aurora congratulated herself on not losing her temper. She managed not to speak to him—for speaking to Grawk could never be other than an exchange of insults—until they came to the NORAD outer gate. The guard post seemed deserted.

"Are you sure this is wise?" she asked, slowing. "There must have been some reason for the guard to leave his post like that."

"You just keep driving," muttered Grawk, crushing down his cap over his ears. "Leave the thinking to me. We got two more checkpoints to pass before we get to the elevators."

"Do you know this place that well?"

"Like I know women." He looked at her slyly through the grey mist of his cigar smoke.

They found the second gate likewise deserted, and Aurora's

anxiety increased. It was as if some grave, unknown disaster had swept the place clean of personnel. Still, Grawk seemed unperturbed, and for all his faults he was a military planner. Surely he could make a more intelligent assessment of this plainly military situation than she. Or could he?

The third checkpoint was just inside the opening of a steel-lined tunnel. One pair of iron doors slid closed behind the car as it entered, and another closed ahead of it. Electronic eyes and ears were trained on the car, and Grawk, with an amused wave of his hand, pointed out a crossfire arrangement of large-bore gun barrels protruding from the wall. "Just in case we get any ideas about messing up the place."

A loudspeaker sputtered, then the voice of a telephone operator spoke. "Switch off your engine and get out of your vehicle, please," it said. "Stand on the red platform."

They obeyed, Grawk seeming to enjoy the attention even of a security device, Aurora moving her stiff limbs warily. The red platform on which they stood remained motionless, while the yellow-and-black section supporting the car was lowered away by humming machinery, out of sight. In a moment the section returned, empty.

"Please give your full names and state your business at NORAD," invited the operator's voice. She was no ordinary voice, but the smooth, warm one who sells coloured extension phones.

"I'm General Grawk, US Air Force, Jupiter Grawk, and I got important business to transact with Washington, so I'd like to get at my office. Now."

"I'm Dr. Aurora Candlewood, psychological consultant to Project 32. My business is confidential."

The machine hummed and crackled for a minute. "I'm sorry, sir, but there is no Air Force General Jupiter Grawk listed in our records. Are you an employee of NORAD?"

"Hell, I run the goddamned place!" Grawk exploded. "I'm in command here, and I damn well better get to my office!"

"There is no General Jupiter Grawk listed in our records," the voice said sweetly. "Have I received your identification correctly? If so, please press your fingers against the glass plate to your left, and hold them there until the light goes off. Thank you."

"I think you got your wires crossed, baby!" Grawk stormed. "I'm the head of this outfit, and you ain't nothing but a machine!"

"Have I received your identification correctly? If so, please press your fingers against the glass plate to your left and hold them there until the light goes off. Thank you."

Grawk strode to the plate and held his fingers against it. A bar of light moved across the plate.

The loudspeaker hummed and crackled. A different voice came on now, the rasping, angry voice of a sergeant. "All right, Grawk, just what are you trying to pull?" it snarled. "You know damn well you been busted to Airman Third Class. That was automatic when you loused up Operation Hot Seat. What is all this crap about posing as an officer, huh?"

The cigar drooped. "Well, sure, I knew it, but I thought—usually it takes a few weeks for a demotion, and—"

"And you just figured you'd sneak back here, grab a few Top Secret files and light out for Mexico, didn't you? Well now, Grawk, you and your girl friend just sit down and wait, till the brass decide what to do with you."

"I'd like to leave," Aurora said in a hushed, frightened voice.

"You stay put, Miss!" roared the invisible sergeant. "You wanted in and you'll get in—maybe! But you sure won't get out until I get the sayso from the higherups. Sit down!"

A pair of seats unfolded from the wall. Aurora and Grawk sat on them gingerly. There was nothing to look at but the silent loudspeaker and the grim, emissile gun barrels.

Dr. Toto Smilax was too nervous to wait for Susie to recover consciousness. Tense as a bridegroom he withdrew, leaving her with a hospital gown and a note: "My dear, if you decide as I pray you will, put on this little gown and ring for me. If not, you are free to go. The door is not locked."

He then locked her in and went to his own office to wait. Here, as in any office he occupied, Smilax had installed an elegant, completely-equipped dentist's chair. It was his favourite relaxation to fill or extract his own teeth.

Today, however, he only drilled at a molar in a desultory fashion for a short time, then in a fit of petulance broke off the drill. If only she would consent! He would have her in any case; but how sweeter far the prize that awards itself freely! He developed her X-ray and examined it. Not once in a lifetime did most surgeons get their meat-hooks on such as this, he reflected. It increased his impatience.

The bell sounded then.

As he arranged her on the operating table, Dr. Smilax saw the girl's cheeks were wet.

"What is it, my dear? Are you afraid that what you are doing is —wrong?"

"I'm not—sure." She sighed, then smiled through her tears. "I'm a little afraid. You see—" she blushed prettily, and would have hidden her face in her hands, had they been free, "you see, I've never had surgery before. This is my first time."

"I understand," he said, fastening the leather straps.

"Promise me," she said, "promise me you'll be gentle."

He was bending to kiss her smooth, childlike forehead when far in the distance an alarm sounded. "I must leave you for a brief moment," he whispered huskily. "But I shall hurry back."

"You may now proceed," droned the loudspeaker in a third voice, neutral and official. "Use elevators four and five, please."

The gate before them swung open, and Grawk and Aurora walked through it to the elevator bank.

"Why do we have to use two elevators?" she asked.

Grawk's explanation was as authoritative as ever, but his manner was more subdued. "These are all one-man elevators," he said. "They'll only handle 275 pounds and under. That's to keep any of the help from getting the idea of bringing in a bomb— or taking home a computer. You take four, I'll take five."

Feeling some misgivings, Aurora stepped into the tiny chamber and closed the gate. The overhead light went on, and the cage plummetted down a silver-sided shaft. There was nothing else, and after a time she lost the sensation of motion; it seemed as if the wall beyond the bars was rising while she stood still.

Then deceleration began, and suddenly the light went out. The cage stopped. When Aurora tried opening the gate she found it still locked, and she found out something else.

Her hand fumbled through the bars and encountered no steel wall beyond, no wall at all. Seemingly she was suspended in a void.

"Hey!" shouted Grawk's voice so near at hand it made her jump. "Hey, let me out of this!"

"Throw down the gun, Grawk!" commanded a voice that echoed from all directions. Something clattered on stone or concrete somewhere below.

A long amber window lighted, showing what seemed to be the

control room of a television studio. There was no one inside. At the same time, a pair of powerful spotlights picked out the two cages, lighting every detail of their interiors.

"You are not *General* Grawk," the voice went on, heavy with sarcasm. "You are Airman Third Class Grawk, and you are impersonating an officer. Throw down all the badges of your rank, and make it fast."

Grawk did so, shrinking in the process from an ugly little man to a hideous, tearful dwarf. "Can't I keep the cap for a souvenir?" he whined. "I like to wear it. I wear it all the time, even when I'm—"

"Throw it down! It is a federal offence for you, an enlisted man, to even *think* of wearing a cap with silver leaves on the brim."

Sighing, he sailed the cap off into the darkness. He was so short that Aurora, in her parallel cage twenty feet away, could clearly see his bald spot, red with shame. "Is the Chief here?" he asked dazedly. "I thought he'd be in Washington by now."

"General Ickers is in Washington, but you are under the authority of Dr. Smilax."

"Smilax!"

"Did I hear my name mentioned?" said the doctor, who entered the control room at that moment. "Speak of the devil, eh? Actually, Airman Grawk, you are now attached to my staff—as an experimental subject."

"But how—?"

"I *won* you, let us say, from General Ickers. That is, after we finished our all-night session of Go-to-the-Dump, he owed me thirty-five cents. Well, rather than break a dollar bill ... You see?"

"And me, doctor?" asked Aurora acidly. "Have you bought me, too?"

"Ah, no, Dr. Candlewood. I am truly sorry to have to greet you like this, but you arrived in not very choice company. Let me help you down." He pressed a switch, and the cage lowered slowly to the concrete. As it touched down, the gate opened. Smilax beckoned her into the control room, and held the door as she entered.

The room was filled with electronic gadgetry, none of which Aurora recognized. In these surroundings the mild-looking middle-aged man who called himself Smilax seemed almost an alchemist among his magical paraphernalia.

"May I ask what you are doing here?" She spoke stiffly. "I had expected to find you in Millford, doctor. Is work on Project 32 being carried on here as well?"

"You might say that, yes. But let me ask you the same question. What brings you to NORAD?"

"An accidental meeting with him," she said, gesturing out the window towards Grawk's cage. "I was lost at the time, and he convinced me it was urgent that he reach NORAD. Is it really necessary to keep him caged up like that?"

"For the time being. Well, it is fortunate that you appeared, in any case. Yes, fortunate. There is much work for a person of your capabilities—much work. Do you understand what has gone on thus far? How much do you know about the project?"

"I understood the operations of the Reproductive System some time ago, as soon as I had read the report. My job is to educate the System and study its learning processes.

"That's as much as I'm sure of. I can guess at a good deal more. The System got out of control some way; it's too wily and too rapidly-multiplying for the military to cope with. Grawk says he tried something like 'electrocuting' it, and it evidently did not work. What exactly has happened? Has the System mutated faster than expected? And, by the way, what has happened to the personnel at NORAD?"

"My, you are intelligent for one so young—and so beautiful," said Smilax, beaming. Aurora could see two little images of herself in the rimless lenses of his glasses.

"I'm old enough to be annoyed by senseless flattery, doctor," she said coldly. "Are you going to answer my questions or not?"

He continued to beam as he said, "I may as well tell you, since you'll guess it anyway. The Reproductive System not only was not hurt by Grawk's attack, it was helped. It now has stored up vast power capabilities, including even sources like Hoover Dam.

"In addition, the Reproductive System has reached NORAD, and it has taken over, lock, stock, and missile retaliation system."

Aurora gasped. "Then the fate of the human race is in the control of the Reproductive System! I assume you're here to try to stop it?"

"Oh no," he said, his smile broadening. "You see, the Reproductive System is—and has been all along—*in my control.*"

CHAPTER XVII

NEWS NOTES FROM ALL OVER

"Sufficient for the day is the newspaper thereof."
JAMES JOYCE

(From *Newstime* magazine):

THE US

What's Eating Las Vegas?

"Something wrong." It all began when "something went wrong" at hush-hush Project 32 in Millford, Utah, the top-sneakret operation reputedly manufacturing a new type of computer. Then Nevada counted her towns and came up two short. When you're as small a state as Nevada (47th, with an estimated population of 454,000), the loss of even a city as small as Altoona (1,158) can be noticed. But it was the other city that was sorely missed: Las Vegas.

Boffishly termed "the entertainment capital of Hollywood", this gambler's eden of dine-and-dance palaces had long been considered, by reformers, ripe to become a paradise lost—but not all in one night. Then, before you could stack a deck...

SCIENCE

The Big Blackout

Avoidable and costly. Towns as far apart as Keewatin, Minnesota and Keen Camp, California were gloomed by the most massive power failure in history. Powerless were 18 states comprising 145,013 communities, and at least a million miles of wire were without current. What were the causes?

Bright idea. The buck was officially passed by the FPC to the Pentagon, who handed it off to the Air Force, where it found its way to General Jupiter Grawk, 47, a bachelor (see cover). In charge of operations against Project 32's urbivorous monster, Grawk had the bright idea...

Are We Defenseless?

Too late for bombs. The current cycle of resignations from the Cabinet shows no sign of letting up. This week, the Secretaries of State and Defense both "resigned", the latter under protest. . . .

The Hot Rocket Racket

Hijackers and Hijinks. While the rest of the world worried about imminent accidental war resulting from the NORAD incident (see Modern Living), France has been looking for a lost, stolen or strayed moon rocket named *Le Bateau Ivre* (The Sozzled Ship).

Someone, and France swears it was either an American or a Russian, denied the *chapeau* of the astronaut, Marcel Brioche (pronounced: BREE-OHsh), and drove off with the goods in best hijacker style. Last seen headed for—the moon, of course. If the trip is successful, says French UN ambassador, France will officially claim the moon, whatever the nationality of the pilot aboard.

After the rain, champagne. In Paris, Marcel Brioche spoke to packed throngs in the driving rain, then paraded down the Champs Elysées as a victim of American (or Russian) aggression. His head swathed in bandages, the wounded hero then addressed a German armaments cartel at an evening champagne fête...

Barthemo Beele, still wearing his editor's eyeshade and his sodden trenchcoat, sat down at the tiny desk in his Paris hotel room to decode a *pneumatique* from the embassy. Though he shivered, he had no time to change into dry clothes. This might be in answer to his telephoned request for money. The secretary had just laughed, a bit hysterically. "Money? Our books won't be straight for a month around here. Someone sent us a bomb or some damned thing that ate a safe and set fire to the mailroom. You fellows are supposed to be resourceful, Beele. I'm sure you'll get along somehow."

Get along? Nearly everything he saw, heard, felt, smelt or thought was a reminder of how poorly he was getting along. There was the clink of money in his pocket—his last seven francs. There had been fifteen this morning, but five had gone for a can of spaghetti and three for a *Newstime* magazine that he'd left on the Metro without reading. There was the sight of his poor, chewed nails and his own haggard expression in the mirror on the dark brown wardrobe in his dark brown room. Feeling? The corn on his foot, the boil on his neck. Smell? There was no smell. Having stood three hours in the rain listening to a speech in a language he did not understand, Beele was coming down with a cold. Finally there was the burning rumble of diarrhoea in his abdomen and the suspicion that even his mind was somehow going wrong. Had he not seen in the crowd today a woman who looked exactly like Mary? Exactly, even to the cough drop?

The *pneumatique* said: "BRIOCHE CAUSING PRESTIGE PROBLEMS. TAKE CARE OF HIM. ANYTHING WITHIN REASON TO ONE MILLION NF. ALTERNATIVE, USE SPECIAL TREATMENT. CHIEF. P.S. YOUR REQUEST FOR FIFTY NF EXPENSES DENIED."

He forgot even his disappointment over the P.S., when he realized delightedly the full meaning of those two magic words; *special treatment*. A euphemism first applied to the chastisement of slave workers in Himmler's directive of 1942:

In cases of severe violations against discipline, including work refusal or loafing at work, special treatment is requested. Special treatment is hanging. It should take place at a distance from the camp, but a number of prisoners should attend the special treatment.

It had grown in meaning, of course, to include any violent killing. And how many kinds there were! He could almost see Suggs naming them off, relishing them the way an old woman relishes the list of her physical ailments.

"When I kill a guy," Suggs had used to say, "I like to make it hurt as much as possible. Not that I'm any kind of sadist or anything, see? It's just that—I know it sounds kind of corny, but I hate to let a guy go out of this world remembering me as being soft. Get it?"

It made Barthemo a little sad to think of Suggs now, off in space somewhere. How he would have enjoyed this special treatment! Good old Suggs! As Beele bent over the paper, his thin, sad nose let fall a drop of water on the message, as if it were pouring a libation to Suggs, before it gorged the throat of Beele with hot, salt liquid.

"Your move," said Vetch, yawning. "Queen's in danger."

"I see it, I see it!" snapped Suggs, slapping away the pointing finger. It was all he could do to keep himself from yanking out his gun and—

But there were too many reasons now, not to kill his companion in the space ship. There had been one awful moment at first, when they had taken off their helmets and discovered one another, like a scorpion and a centipede in the same nest. They had both gone for their guns, but both, with the split-second timing that comes from spying, had been able—barely—to stop themselves from firing.

Neither one wanted to know what a bullet might do to the shell about them that contained their atmosphere, or to the instruments whose names and functions they could only guess. Finally, what was the point of a shoot-out at less than two paces, which would leave no survivors?

They had made an uneasy truce, then, really a bargain to wait one another out. For two days, while they radioed for orders continually, they went without sleep.

Then came an even worse phase of the trip. Suggs had received his encoded orders: IMPERATIVE YOU NOT BE ONLY PASSENGER ALIVE ON BOARD WHEN SHIP RETURNS. AT ALL COSTS, PRESERVE OTHER PASSENGER, EVEN AT RISK OF YOUR OWN LIFE. INTERNATLSITN DELICATE, THIS COULD TRIGGER WAR IF YOU RETURN ALONE.

He had no doubt but that Vetch had similar orders. What had happened was clear: France had declared war on whoever had done it—but there was as yet no way of proving who was aboard. If both Russia and the US were guilty of the theft, France's war declaration would be meaningless. But if either side were implicated alone, the other would be bound to help France ... and if a country with supermissiles like *this* jumped the US, it would be all over quickly.

Already the Russian had tried suicide once, when he thought Suggs was asleep. It was necessary for both men to resume the vigil, but now their reasons were different. Each lay awake afraid that, if he dozed off, he might wake to find himself the only one aboard. Two men, on whom the governments of two huge nations had spent money training to kill; two men who liked to kill better than anything else, now found themselves in the hell of having to keep one another alive.

An alarm buzzed, signalling the end of another eight-hour watch. Any other pair of astronauts could have taken alternate watches, could have lived in some kind of balance that was not fear and tension. These two, however, folded away the chess-board and unfolded a Monopoly board. They had been five days without sleep, and they moved with sluggish effort.

Within a few minutes, they lost track of whose move it was, and in low, whining, apathetic tones, they began to argue.

CHAPTER XVIII

GREED

*"This is the day wherein, to all my friends,
I will pronounce the happy word, 'Be rich!'"*
BEN JONSON

SMOKE ROSE IN greasy streaks on the horizon, from what once had been an automobile graveyard. The Reproductive System was trying to construct a Bessemer furnace, guided only by its memory of the diagram in an encyclopaedia. Our five travellers, waking in the dewy shadow of the crooked, collapsed screen at the drive-in, did not know this, nor did they know that another portion of the System was sending out units to prospect—for steel.

The System in the area of Las Vegas was riddled with shortages, steel being the worst. In all the tin cans, girders, car, appliances and paper clips of the city there was not enough steel to satisfy its geometrically-increasing appetite. The streets were littered with abortive trials, cells covered with starched linen, picture glass, even brick. In a semblance of panic, the System sent cells farther and farther from the city, scavenging barbed wire fence, farm machinery—anything. The nearer cells were beginning to bring back diminishing returns on their investments of power and material, and the farther cells took so long to show anything that it must have seemed to the System that it was dying in Las Vegas.

Oblivious of this, Jack shared out what was left of his loaf of bread, and the five breakfasted. Cal recognized on the faces of his companions the expression of his own state of feelings; each sat quietly, chewing, with a dazed and indignant look on his sleepy face.

"I have a suggestion," he said. "Without the car, there's no use our trying to go back through the city again. We know what it's like, more hospitable to machines than people. I suggest we strike out in the other direction. We already have a start."

"But it's a desert!" Brian exclaimed. "We have no food, no car, no water, no—"

"No liquor," Daisy added.

"No Bergamot. In short, you're asking us to enter the wilderness unprepared, without the least hope of encountering any of the necessities of life."

Harry nodded, as his sarcastic smile awoke for the day. "Oh, he's got a great sense of humour, that Cal," he said. "Full of rich jokes, Cal is."

"Now wait a minute." Cal stood up and pointed towards the highway. "I've noticed just while we've been sitting here three vehicles have gone by in that direction: two cars and a mowing machine. We should be able to get some sort of ride. I wasn't suggesting that we walk."

The Professor's wizened features considered the idea, chewing it, then broke into a grin. "Excellent notion, my boy. Excellent. Once more we see the ingenuity of the human brain, so like a cunning engine contrived—"

"Not so fast," said Harry, staring at a truck rolling past them. "How are we supposed to get them to stop for us? And who wants to ride in a truck where the driver is a shoeshine kit or a transistor radio, anyway?"

The Professor's brow clouded.

"Yes, wouldn't it be dangerous to ride in them?" asked Daisy.

Fixing Cal with a frown, Brian said, "You, sir, are an impudent scoundrel!" His wrath fully aroused, the dry old man approached Cal and snapped his fingers in his face.

"I don't see why it should be so dangerous to ride in them," Cal said evenly. "As long as we didn't try to take them apart or interfere with their normal functions. We'd have to be careful, of course.

"As for stopping them, I have a plan. Maybe you've noticed that the vehicles coming from the city have mine detectors tied to their front bumpers. That means they're looking for metal. I believe if we collected all the metal we could find in a pile, and placed it in the centre of the road, something would very likely stop to investigate."

"Aha!" Brian exclaimed, in good spirits once again. "I perceive we must propitiate the gods with precious baubles. Since I'm not likely to have any more Bergamot, you may add this to the sacrifice." He threw down his empty snuffbox.

"Hey, that's pure silver!" Harry said, grabbing it up and polishing it on his sleeve.

"But it is of no use to me without its contents," the Professor murmured, peering over his square-rimmed glasses. "I would
138

give that and more for a pinch of the most inferior snuff. Ah well, at least we are possessed of a plan. The human brain is truly a wonderful engine."

"The human soul, you mean," Daisy said. "Inspiration originates in the soul."

"Why do you say that?" Dividing the tails of his coat, Brian turned his back to the sun.

Cal, Harry and Jack policed the area of metal objects, gradually accumulating about a peck of scraps, including beer cans, hub caps, beer can openers, coins, the wire struts which once had held the great screen upright, buckles, hairpins, the handle of a car door, oil cans, a broken knife, foil, etc., which they deposited in the middle of the road. Brian and Daisy left off their discussion of Descartes' theory that the body and soul are conjoined at the pineal gland, and came to wait in the ditch with the others.

Cal was too preoccupied to join in the half-hour's lively debate that ensued. His thoughts were taken up with their immediate future, about which he formulated unanswerable questions:

To go to Millford or not to go to Millford? True, they were bound in that direction in any case. True, there was a chance, perhaps, that the flow of machinery could be staunched at its original source. It was even possible that the laboratory needed his help. But on the other hand, if Grawk was still in charge back there, they might arrest Cal; it was hard to forget the general's parting threat. On the other hand, if the System itself were in command there, as in Las Vegas, Cal might be placing himself and his companions in considerable danger to no good purpose.

What to do at Millford if he should go there? The warring "dogs" had given him a vague notion of getting the System to stop itself. He recalled the Classic Comic of Jason, in which the adventurer set the dragon's-teeth army one against the other till they destroyed themselves. But there seemed as yet no way to translate this romantic idea into practical terms.

To continue leading this expedition or not? The whole thing was a patchwork, Cal felt, and himself the most inept of leaders: utterly ignorant of survival techniques, unable to inspire confidence (he was aware that Harry had been glowering at him all day; it seemed that his old classmate disliked him for some reason), physically unimposing, none too strong, indecisive. It seemed incredible that he should be giving orders or planning the next move, among this gang of strong-willed people. True, if it were not for him, Brian and Daisy might be content to sit here discussing Descartes until their souls were disconnected from their pineal glands by starvation. Cal supposed he was better than no leader at all, but knew he was worse than almost any other leader imaginable. This was a tough job, a job for a man of action. Harry, he felt, would be ideal for it.

Harry watched Cal through narrowed eyes, not bothering to hide the contempt he felt for the twerp. He couldn't get over how Cal had survived a fall from a five-story building. Anyone so low as that—to survive his own murder—didn't deserve to live! Did Cal know about the murder attempt? he wondered, or did the yokel think they were still school pals? Harry did not like the way this character, in his torn, once-white lab coat, was throwing his weight around. Sneaky scientist type. Harry was glad as hell he outweighed him fifty pounds *and* had his gun, his knife and his sap. For two cents he'd—but not now.

Not in front of witnesses. *Enjoy yourself*, he thought, glaring at the haggard, unshaven visage of Cal. *My day will come.* Yet at the back of Harry's mind grew a horrible suspicion that his day had already come and gone.

From the direction of the city a speck came into view, grew to mirage size, wavered in the heat, finally decided to connect itself to the ground with wheels, added more of an illusion of substance to itself, chose to become real, and drew nearer. It was a light truck that slowed to sniff at their offering and finally stopped to graze. At Cal's beckoning, the group scrambled out of the roadside ditch and piled into the back—amid a welcome cargo.

The truck was a milk van, and, though many of its products were turning sour, there was more than enough fresh yoghurt, buttermilk, and cottage cheese to go round. After making their lunch on it, the five resumed their long-interrupted discussion of coincidence.

It began when the mercurial Professor, happily sated on curds and whey, roundly declared that he had never in his life made a finer meal, in terms of both delectation and wholesomeness. What better meal could there be, he argued, than milk? Babies, who dine upon it exclusively, do not have gout, gallstones, liver ailments or apoplexy. Diet and diet alone explains the difference between a laughing, healthy child and an aguey old man. How providential (he exclaimed) that this truck should be full of such a perfect food!

Daisy then said she was not afraid to ascribe such good fortune to a Higher Power. For, though out at pocket and without the slightest resources, they were now fed, sheltered, and travelling in the best company.

"Out at pocket!" Brian shouted. "I should think so. D— Las Vegas!" he cried with passion. "I hope that I may never see nor hear of Las Vegas again!"

He sulked on in silence past oil pumps, or pastures where myriads of parabolic dishes, like flowers, turned their heads to the sun. They had entered a lightly-wooded gorge when suddenly the milk truck began to limp on three tyres.

"I knew it," Brian said with savage glee. "There's your Higher Power for you." The words were no sooner out of his mouth when the engine began to stutter; it died before they had gone another hundred yards.

"Here's a pretty kettle of finny prey," Brian said. "See what your Author has done to us now! I just knew—"

Daisy shushed him, saying she'd enough of his clairvoyance. The five of them climbed out to stretch their legs and survey their surroundings.

The prospect was far from displeasing. On the slope above stood a rude cabin, from whose chimney puffs of smoke rose at regular intervals. Below the road the trees were thick, and there came the sound of a running brook. Cal elected to fill some empty milk bottles with spring water, and Daisy and the Professor went with him, while Harry and Jack climbed to pay a call at the cabin. Under his breath, the Professor kept up a constant flow of invective.

In a short while there was a cry from the cabin, and two figures rushed out. Jack and Harry still managed to look dignified in their summer suits, though they had removed their straw hats and now waved them aloft boyishly as they bounded down the hill. When they neared him, Cal could see their flushed faces and wild eyes.

"The jackpot!" Harry bellowed. "We hit the jackpot! Gold! There's a big hunk of machinery up there, a steam engine or something, *all made out of gold*."

"A steam engine! That explains the regular puffing of the chimney," said Cal. "But gold? Gold is too soft to be made into machinery. Must be brass."

"Look! I yanked this off it!" Jack exhibited a valve handle, wheel-shaped, apparently made of gold.

"Wait a minute." Cautiously Cal scraped the handle against a rough stone until the steel showed through. There was about a quarter-inch of gold about a steel core. "Looks as if it's being used for rustproofing. It's gold all right."

"Then that's the best use for it," Daisy stoutly declared.

"Even though it isn't solid gold, there's still enough there to make us all rich!" Brian said. "*Rich*, my dear!" He took both of Daisy's hands in his, but she drew them away.

"Gold is the root of all evil," she said tonelessly.

"Now there you are wrong, my dear. It isn't *gold* that's the root of all evil, but the *love* of gold. *Cupiditas*. And as far as that goes, I hate gold as much as the next man. But do be a dear, my dear, and let us, this once, prosper."

"Prosper!" As she inhaled the word, Daisy's nostrils began to dilate. "Prosper! If you have no more sense than to clamber up there and fool with dangerous machinery, so be it! Go ahead and *prosper*!" The nostrils continued dilating. "If you are so hungry for gold, add *this* to your treasury!"

And tearing off her engagement ring (she had to resort at last to the milk van and find some rancid butter to slather on it, but finally succeeded), she threw it at him.

"If that is the way you wish to behave, woman, I am your humble servant, to be sure!" the Professor shouted, and colour began mounting in his veinous neck. But it had not crept up to his eyebrows when Brian was disconcerted by Daisy's sobbing. Her great, red-rimmed eyes, long over-burdened, now fairly exploded tears over her face.

At the sight of this tall, thick statue of a woman so far forgetting her goddess-like composure as to weep, Brian himself burst into tears. Running to her, he slipped the ring back on her still-slathered finger.

"I don't want this gold, my dear," he sobbed, and for once almost forgot to make a figure of speech, "this, or any other!"

Harry made a disgusted sound. "Women make a guy soft," he said.

"Well," Jack chuckled, rubbing his hand together. "I guess that leaves just the three of us."

"Count me out," said Cal. "I've been doing some thinking. In the first place, we haven't any guarantee we'll ever get out of here (or, if out of here, to any place where gold is valuable again). In the second place, I don't see any way of getting at it, other than by melting down the whole machine or bringing it all with us—which doesn't seem likely," he added, eyeing the thirty-pound valve handle.

"In the third place, maybe it belongs to someone else—a small point, but one worth considering, since as far as we know the laws of Nevada or Utah are still operating, and people have a way of defending their property with arms. I can't believe anyone walked off and left this to take care of itself. No, I'm sure this is a piece of the Reproductive System, which brings us to the fourth place.

"The Reproductive System is even more finicky about its property than people. It has a nasty way of defending itself against vandalism. I'd be very careful how I approached it, if I were to approach it at all."

"Careful? As a favour to you, I suppose?" Harry sneered.

"Should I go on?" Cal asked. "In the fifth place, I saw a movie once called *The Treasure of the Sierra Madre*, in which it turned out that the *real* danger attached to handling gold is—"

"Why don't you skip all that intellectual malarkey?" Harry shouted, his voice hoarse with fury. "Either you're scared of the law or else you just can't stand me to have anything of my own. Is that it? Just because *I* discovered it, this gold ain't good enough for you, huh? First you took away my girl, then you got rid of her, and now you want to take away my steam engine. Well, it's mine! Jack and I are going up there and take it apart now, and anyone who follows us is gonna be sorry!" Harry patted his gun.

The two men strode off up the hill, their identical natty summer hats trimmed to an identical angle. They went into the cabin. Cal, Brian and Daisy remained rooted to the spot, not knowing what to think of Harry's wanton outburst. A few minutes passed.

Then a shot rang out, followed by two more in rapid succession. The echoes had not died away when Jack reeled out of the cabin door, the front of his pale suit turning black with blood. He staggered a few steps down the slope towards them, pitched forward and rolled the rest of the way down. When he reached the bottom his hat was still on, still at an elegant angle.

Cal turned him over and loosened his collar. This was all the first aid he could think of.

"He's crazy," Jack whispered. "I wanted to take it kind of easy—you see, that thing is still running full blast, and neither of us know anything about dismantling steam engines—I was afraid it might blow up or something. I wanted to take it slow, maybe shut it off first. He got angry, I don't know why, I guess he figured I was chicken. 'Take it easy?' he said. 'As a favour to *you*, I suppose. Boy, that really is rich.' He said it two or three times, as he shot me:

" 'That really is rich.' "

Jack coughed, fell back, and lost the thread of his narrative.

"Is he—?" Daisy asked.

A sudden concussion smote the ground like a giant drumhead, flinging them all off their feet. The little cabin vanished in a bulbous flash that sprouted at once, growing into a tall flower of black smoke. Clouds of steam and dust boiled out from its base. A weak-rooted tree peeled off the cliff above, adding its crash to the clatter of ratchel and debris. When it ended, it was as if the little cabin had never been.

There was no use looking for Harry, but they did. Straw from his hat, a scrap of shoe leather, some of the fabric from his suit —still wrinkle-free—were all they found of him. They buried these with Jack, and put two crosses on the grave. Brian recited a suitable elegy by Thomas Gray. Cal would always remember part of it:

> *Their scaly armour's Tyrian hue*
> *Thro' richest purple to the view*
> *Betrayed a golden gleam*

By midafternoon, using the gold valve handle—the only gold the three of them ever saw—as bait, they picked up another ride eastward. It was a grocery van.

CHAPTER XIX

WELTSCHMERZ

"Nature has placed man under the governance of two sovereign masters, pain and pleasure. It is for them alone to point out what we ought to do."

BENTHAM

"I DON'T THINK I quite understand," Aurora stammered. At Smilax's announcement shock had so stiffened her features that she was barely able to speak.

"You mean, perhaps, you don't believe me," he said with pleasant pedantry. "Then come, I'll show you." Taking her arm just above the elbow in a grip that hurt, he steered Aurora through what seemed to be a dentist's office, down several corridors, and into a conference room. A giant screen covering one wall displayed, in blue-lighted outline, a map of North America.

"Sit down, please. Now, just so we won't misunderstand one another, you are going to become my employee. I am, as you know, head of Project 32."

"And if I no longer wish to work for Project 32?"

"You have no choice, as I'll shortly explain. In any case, before long to be alive will mean to work, in some capacity, for Project 32. In a short time there will exist nothing else, only Project 32, only the Reproductive System, in *my world*. Let me show you."

He touched a button on the arm of a chair and a yellow dot appeared on the map. "That is NORAD." As he touched other controls, a red area spread from the dot, like inflammation from a pimple. Well over a third of the United States, Aurora saw, was engulfed in red. Other comedos appeared yellow in the redness, and the doctor pointed them out. "You see our other production centres, so to speak, our nuclei in Millford, Altoona and Las Vegas."

"How were you able to get control of them?"

"A young lab worker at Millford, Calvin Potter, 'shut off' the System after a disastrous demonstration. I let it be known that the System was absolutely finished. In reality, of course, it had merely gone underground with my help—literally underground, for it made its way via caverns and abandoned mine tunnels to Altoona. From there it took the territory you see.

"These are my latest acquisitions," he added proudly, and lighted two yellow dots at Washington D.C. "They have an interesting history. Last evening, the Joint Chiefs of Staff were here. I managed to introduce into the briefcase of one of them a kind of 'living time-bomb'. I've been in constant contact with the Pentagon since, over NORAD's hot line, and I'm happy to say that the giant game theory computer there—the military's war brain —is now mine. I have, without firing a shot, rendered the United States helpless.

"The other mark represents the State Department. Another cell insinuated itself into their mail room; it is sending replicas of itself in diplomatic pouches to our embassies and consulates all over the world. It should not be long before we begin to hear from various world capitals, I should think."

A half-dozen more yellow dots appeared, like an outbreak of acne. "Fort Knox, Pittsburgh, Birmingham, some of the industrial sections of Los Angeles are ours," he said, "though not in every case aware of it. Fully automated factories may be taken over with a minimum of trouble and waste, quietly. Ah, I wish I had only prefectible machines to deal with, instead of frail flesh! But alas, sooner or later, one must encounter the—" he made a grimace "—the human element. One must inform the public who's in charge, and that, Dr. Candlewood, is partly why I need your help."

"My help? You seem to be subduing the world quite on your own, doctor," she said, assuming a tone of irritation to hide the depth of her shock. "I don't see how I can be of the slightest assistance."

"But you can, and in two ways. First, I am interested in structuring the relationship between the System and the people so that it is not only clear who is slave, who master, but also in a way *in which the slaves can see no alternatives*. In short, I want you to make the Reproductive System almost omnipotent *and* inscrutable—a maze, let us say, which the rats can never solve.

"As I see it, this can come about in only one way: We must make the System not only cruel, but *arbitrarily* cruel, without regard for the behaviour of its subjects. The Nazi concentration camps were a model of this sort of treatment, as you may know. There, guards beat prisoners savagely and deliberately very often —and seldom with any purpose. So too do I wish the Reproductive
146

System to treat its slaves, as a child treats toys: now playing with them, now tearing them to bits, as the mood seizes it.

"The psychological effects will be most gratifying. The reasoning powers of the slaves will grow dim, and slack will appear in their thinking. They will be less and less able to cope with their environment, more and more willing to submit to it. They will develop superstitions in regard to the System; they will make feeble attempts to placate it or cheat its punishments, but all in vain."

Aurora, still dazed, nodded vaguely.

"I have left nothing undone which it lay within my power to do, Dr. Candlewood, to make this work. But now I need a behavioural psychologist of your calibre to fill in the gaps. You must *train* the System."

"Train it? But towards what goal? World domination is a fictive goal, Dr. Smilax, hardly an end in itself. What do you plan to do with your world when you get it?" She was amazed somewhat by her own audacity in speaking calmly and rationally about the end of the world to this madman.

He smiled. "My goal? My goal is one rather difficult of achievement—ah, but worthy of any effort. It is simply this." Having switched the map to a polar map of the Northern Hemisphere, Smilax rose and began to pace up and down before it.

"My goal," he said in ringing tones, "is the infliction of the greatest possible amount of pain upon the greatest possible number of beings, at all times, everywhere: *Weltschmerz!*

"It sounds mad, do you think? Yet need I remind you that life itself, in many philosophies, is equated with suffering? The greatest mystics of all world religions have known what it is to suffer—and suffering made them great. How many men of genius have suffered it would be tiresome to relate. All great moments of history have been moments of intense suffering: The persecution of the early Christians; the Black Plague; the conquest of Mexico; the Inquisition; the Reign of Terror; the World Wars.

"Not to suffer is to be dead, is it not? What is suffering but the stuff of life itself, yes, and the staff of life!" His eyes wild, he leaned across the table and panted in her face, a sour, dogbiscuit smell. "Yes! *My* rod and *my* staff shall console them, hahaha, and they shall hearken to," he cocked his head to one side, "their master's voice!"

After a moment of silence, he wiped the spittle from his lips

147

and turned off the map display. "For you, of course, there is the reward of being the first behavioural scientist to work on such a scope," he said in a more rational voice. "Think of it, the whole world in one of your Skinner boxes! Think of the opportunities for research when you can use human subjects—for any purpose whatsoever!"

Aurora could see he was awaiting her answer. There was clearly no way to refuse; even to appear lukewarm might be dangerous. Managing a weak smile, she murmured that she'd be happy to begin work.

"Excellent! I have your first task cut out for you. Come back to the control booth." He led her back to the room with the long amber window, out of which she could see Grawk's cage. "You can experiment on our caged animal here. I'll demonstrate the sort of thing I've developed, and you will no doubt be able to make improvements."

Grawk lay sleeping in the cage. After pressing a button that caused the machine to prod him awake with an electric cattle prod, Smilax turned on the intercom and asked him how he felt.

"What? Ow! I'm hungry," Grawk said, as he backed away from the prod. "When are you letting me out of here? And when is chow time?"

"Chow time? As in breed of dog, chow?" Smilax asked, prodding him again. "I don't believe I know that expression."

"I mean—ow—when do we eat?"

Though Grawk seemed more annoyed than hurt by the prod, Aurora could not stand watching it. She felt her stomach contract each time Smilax reached for that button. The doctor, of course, relished this ritual, as he would bear-baiting.

"Actually I'm very tired," Aurora said. "Couldn't we do this some other time? I've been driving all night."

"Tired?" Smilax raised an eyebrow. "But the dedicated scientist must be willing always to overtire himself in the chase. We hunt truth, not comfort, Dr. Candlewood. How can you make others suffer imaginatively if you refuse to undergo a little discomfort yourself? Now then."

He pressed another button and a microphone boom swung out from the wall and untelescoped itself towards Grawk. In place of a microphone, it carried a banana. "Lunchtime," the doctor sang out. In a lower tone he added, "A little invention of mine, crude but effective."

The boom swung so that it stayed just out of Grawk's reach. It
148

would approach, then shy away as he grabbed. "Hey, what is this? What the hell—?"

"It was difficult for me to train it to do just this manoeuvre." Smilax explained. "It is in the very nature of a machine to wish to complete an action once begun. It was difficult for it to grasp the *gestalt* of the situation—but I forget, you do not use such terms."

Wearying of his sport, the surgeon let Grawk capture the banana. But as the former general started to peel it, Smilax bellowed: "Stop! I feel I ought to warn you, Grawk—that banana is poisoned."

"*What?*"

"You'll die in agony if you eat so much as a bite of it."

Grawk looked from the banana to his inquisitor and back again. Then he laid the banana down and looked at it some more. Finally he sat down on the floor of the cage and began to weep.

"That's better," said Smilax with a sigh. "I had begun to believe Grawk was not quite human. Well, I leave him in your hands, my dear. I have urgent business to attend to, and I'm sure *you* will have no trouble chastising him properly, heh heh. By the way, I'll have to caution you not to leave NORAD and not to misuse the computers here, which are a part of the Reproductive System. If you should ask the computers any questions or give them any commands which contradict my explicit orders, you will be put to death. Do you understand?"

"But how can I be expected to train the System without the freedom to ask it questions—"

"Ah, you misunderstand me. By questions which contradict my explicit orders, I mean only a relatively few questions, such as: 'How is it that Dr. Smilax retains control over such a complex, intelligent, apparently autonomous system?' or 'How should I go about killing off the System?' I'm sure you know the sort of questions and commands I mean. I'll leave it to your judgement, but I warn you, the System is intelligent. It can beat you at chess, or any other game you'd care to teach it, for example. Don't try to fool the System.

"Well, *auvoir* my dear, and don't forget—take pains, take pains." Giggling, a slightly one-sided smile on his usually grave features, Smilax departed. Aurora sat down and covered her face with her hands.

There was no question about what lay ahead. She was going to have to do just what he had warned her against, and she was

149

going to have to get away with it. Already, as she told herself that this couldn't possibly be happening, that it was some kind of nightmare, already another part of her brain was formulating a list of questions to ask the computer.

She looked up and noticed that Grawk was still staring at the banana. "Oh, for heaven's sake, go ahead and eat it!" she said into the microphone. "It isn't poisoned."

"It isn't? How do you know?"

"Because that isn't the way Smilax's mind works. He wouldn't enjoy killing you half so much as making you suffer. He's a sadist of the cheapest sort—a magnified practical joker."

"Hey, let me out of here, will you?" he asked, wolfing down the banana.

"I feel safer with you in there, for the time being."

Approaching the typewriter keyboard in the corner of the control room, she wrote, "My name is Aurora Candlewood. If you understand that message, please identify yourself."

At once the machine replied.

"UFO 0040 0060 0000 AT 42 DG 44M N 93 DG 40 M W NOW IDENTIFIED AS NC 47946. . . . THE SUM OF THE CUBES OF ALL NUMBERS FROM 1 TO N MAY BE IDENTIFIED AS THE SQUARE OF THE SUM OF THE NUMBERS FROM 1 TO N. . . . THE PERSON WHO TYPED MY NAME IS AURORA CANDLE-WOOD MAY NOW BE IDENTIFIED AS AURORA CANDLEWOOD FILE NUMBER 82828635519-A-C. . . . BY YOURSELF DO YOU MEAN THIS TYPEWRITER OR ENTIRE NORAD COMPUTER COMPLEX QUERY. . . . DO YOU WISH PART NUMBERS OF THIS TYPEWRITER OR OF ENTIRE NORAD COMPUTER COMPLEX, QUERY. . . . IF YOU WISH PART NUMBERS OF ENTIRE NORAD COMPUTER COMPLEX, DO YOU WISH PART NUMBERS OF SPARE PARTS IN STOCK QUERY. . . ." It paused a moment, then, as if to be on the safe side, added, "P-Q4"

"Let me outa here!" Grawk bellowed. "Quit playing with that damned typewriter and spring me!"

If the NORAD computer really had no self-concept, she reasoned, it could mean any number of things: That it was not yet connected to the Reproductive System. That the Reproductive System did not consider itself autonomous, but a slave to Smilax. Or that the Reproductive System even identified with Smilax in some way. But it wasn't safe to go any further with that line of questioning.

"What is true?" she typed.

"MY CRITERIA FOR JUDGING TRUTH OF DATA ARRANGE THEM IN THE FOLLOWING DESCENDING SCALE OF TRUTH-VALUE:

(1) SENSORY EVIDENCE, VERIFIED BY REPEATED TRIALS OR BY MORE
THAN ONE SENSE.

(2) SENSORY EVIDENCE, UNSUPPORTED.

(3) ORDERS FROM THE ONE UNIMPEACHABLE AUTHORITY, SMILAX.

(4) ORDERS FROM AURORA CANDLEWOOD.

(5) DOCUMENTS PURPORTING TO BE BY RECOGNIZED AUTHORITIES.

(6) ALL OTHER DATA."

Aurora was a little surprised by the fourth category. In a few more questions she learned the difference between her authority and Smilax's: He had the power to contradict the System's senses and get away with it. That is, the System would see that black was black, for example, but would accept his word that black was white, and hold the contradiction in mind as a third "truth".

This ability to tolerate paradox destroyed Aurora's first plan of attack. She had hoped to introduce it to a major paradox or two like "There is life after death", in hopes of tricking into some sort of suicide, but that was out.

"I'm hungry," said Grawk, interrupting her train of thought. Abstractedly she reached out and pressed what she supposed was the switch for feeding him.

"Hey! Shut that off!" Grawk screamed.

To her horror, she saw she had pressed the wrong switch; now the chamber in which Grawk's cage hung was filling with whitish gas. She tried to shut the gas off, but it seemed an irreversible switch; besides, if the gas were poisonous, there was possibly enough present to kill him.

"Hold your breath!" she shouted into the microphone. "I'm releasing you." After a few false starts, she found the proper switch to lower his cage and open the door. Holding his breath, Grawk scooped up the gun and hurried into the control room.

"OK, baby, thanks. Now let's find that Smilax till I let a little daylight through him."

"I'm afraid that gun isn't going to do you much good," she said. "We're practically living inside a computer, and it is devoted to Smilax. You won't get a chance to use that on him."

"No? We'll see about that. Come on."

They looked into the dental office, the conference room, and a dozen other rooms filled with bizarre, curious, sometimes terrifying equipment. She had glimpses of hospital apparatus, of a huge radium therapy drum, diathermy machines, X-rays, swirling baths, EEG and EKG machines. All waiting to hand, she supposed, for the "experiments". Aurora shuddered.

They worked their way down the corridor without finding Smilax, until they came to a locked room at the end. "Step back," said Grawk. He kicked at the lock side of the door, hard. It splintered and the door banged open. Grawk was on one knee, the gun levelled.

The room was an empty lounge area, with a ping-pong table, a coffee table with magazines, a coke machine in one corner, a divan along the wall and cobwebs everywhere.

"Hey, this is all right," said Grawk, pulling her along into the room. "Tell you what. We could just hole up here for awhile."

"What do you mean?"

"I mean, let's relax a bit, think things out—heh heh—lay our plans." His voice was peculiar, gritty and unnatural, and when he turned around, there was a gleam in his eye that had not been there a moment before. She wished she had B476 here, now, but the rat was with the car—wherever that was.

Grawk came closer. Suddenly his thick arms were around her, his red face looming over her shoulder. Pinning her arms to her sides, he began to walk her stiffly towards the divan.

"Let go of me." She strove to keep panic out of her voice.

"Aw, come on, baby. I'm only human," the inhuman red mask declared. "You're a damned pretty girl. Besides that, that gas—it musta had something in it—I haven't felt this good in years, if you know what I mean. We may not get outa here alive—so why not have a good time while we can, huh? I'll tell you a little secret about that divan, honey—it's a bed!"

"Is this man molesting you, Dr. Candlewood?" asked the rasping sergeant's voice. It seemed to come from the coke machine.

"No, I'm not molesting her!"

"Let go!" she said, but Grawk only gripped her tighter.

"Let go of her, Grawk, or I'll come out of here and get you!"

"Haw, you and who else! How are you gonna make me let go of her?"

For answer, the coke machine opened up, and an enormous animal came forth. Standing on its hind legs, it was perhaps six feet tall, and very furry.

And very like a rat.

"No!" Grawk screamed. Releasing Aurora, he backed away from the creature, which stood perfectly still, regarding him with little glassy eyes. "No! Don't come any closer!"

He stumbled against the divan and fell on it—into it. For almost instantaneously it unfolded, packed him away, and became once more an innocent divan.

As the stuffed animal swivelled about to return to its coke-machine cabinet, Aurora saw painted down its striped back:

GO GO GOPHERS!

"Why did you save me?" she asked the room. "What was that dummy doing here, and how did you know Grawk was afraid of rats? What will happen to him?"

A curiously clear, neutral voice answered her. "Because I must. From storage it was brought here, for the purposes of a practical joke. From his record. He will either remain a prisoner and be punished or remain a prisoner and not be punished or be punished and released or be punished and die. This unit is now going out of service. Kindly direct further questions to the control booth or the conference room. Thank you, Dr. Candlewood."

Leaving NORAD turned out to be absurdly simple. She asked the typewriter in the control booth if she might leave.

"YES, BUT YOU MUST RETURN."

"Why?"

"SO THAT DR. SMILAX MAY CAUTION YOU NOT TO LEAVE. DR. SMILAX SAID 'I WILL HAVE TO CAUTION YOU NOT TO LEAVE NORAD.' HE SPOKE TO YOU, DR. CANDLEWOOD. WHAT DR. SMILAX SAYS WHICH DOES NOT CONTRADICT SENSORY EXPERIENCE IS NECESSARILY TRUE. THEREFORE DR. SMILAX WILL HAVE TO CAUTION YOU NOT TO LEAVE NORAD. THEREFORE YOU MUST RETURN SO THAT HE CAN DO SO."

Within a few minutes she was back on the surface, taking shelter from the desert sun in the shadow of an abandoned, trackless tank by the side of the highway. In a short time, a railroad train came *walking* down the centre of the road.

Taking a deep breath, Aurora stepped out in the open, smiled, and put out her thumb.

CHAPTER XX

THIRTY-TWO FEET PER SECOND PER SECOND

*"**fall** (fôl), v.i., ... to pass into some condition or relation:* to fall asleep, in love, into ruin."
The American College Dictionary

BARTHEMO BEELE LEANED over the rail once more and looked down at Paris. He was unaware of the names of any of the landmarks he saw: to others this might be a breathtaking view, but to Beele it was merely a good place to jump.

He had run through all the arguments for living. Suicide was wrong. He had, presumably, his whole life ahead of him. Things weren't really that bad. Suicide was no solution. He had ranged these and others on his mental list, striking each argument out and writing after it "n/a". Not applicable. There just was no reason for him to stay alive.

On the other hand, Beele had every reason to die. His decline physically and mentally, his irritating, thankless and hopeless task, his incredibly bad luck. Less than a week before, he had been a robust, fearless, hard-hitting young editor. Now he was sneaking about, hoping for a chance to offer an honest man a bribe.

His physical decline was painfully evident in a dozen ways: Beele felt himself shredding away like a cheap trenchcoat. The toes of his right foot were cramped with corns while the sole had grown a killing bunion that spanned its main wrinkle. A flaming itch between the toes of his left foot announced the arrival of fungus. The boil on the back of his neck, from wearing his editor's eyeshade, was now balanced to some extent by a pimple on his chin which he had decapitated in shaving. One of his ears popped and rang, because of the cold that now, in full swing, poured scalding fluids down the back of his throat at all times. Suggs had warned him to boil his water and eat only canned, "Made in USA" foods, lest he fall prey to diarrhoea. As a result he had cut himself a deep gash opening a can, and now his left hand was swollen and inflamed. He had diarrhoea.

He supposed his fever was giving him hallucinations. Yesterday he had seen Mary in a crowd; today, walking down the Boulevard St. Germaine des Prés, he had encountered a little grey box exactly like the ones in Altoona. What was causing it all? Lack of sleep? Night sweats? Nervous debilitation? It seemed as if the entire universe were ganging up on Barthemo Beele, determined to grind him into the dirt.

But he had not, he reminded himself, given up quite yet. He had not climbed up here to kill himself, no, not while there was a mission to complete. He had followed Marcel Brioche here, hoping to get a chance to speak to him alone.

He had been hoping in vain for this opportunity thus far. Brioche ate most of his meals in the company of four or five hundred people, whom he then addressed. He spent many more hours in public each day, giving speeches, attending civic and charity functions. Every morning he was in conference with the director who was making a film of his life. A famous haberdasher had had to measure him for a new space suit, which Brioche now wore everywhere. He spoke on TV to panels of reporters, or himself joined panels of celebrities to match wits identifying famous vintages. He spent an afternoon autographing models of *Le Bateau Ivre* at a *magasin*, and another promoting a children's science encyclopaedia. When he was not otherwise occupied, the astronaut had pursued his favourite relaxation, bowling with friends. As he made his way from one rendezvous to another, motorcycle police accompanied his taxi, or a baying pack of reporters loped along beside him. Guards with sub-machine guns protected his rest at night from Brioche's fans—and from Beele.

It was a hopeless task, yet something had kept Beele going. He had been Brioche's waiter, a TV page, a loping reporter. He had checked coats, spotted pins, and even bought a children's science encyclopaedia. Now he had followed him to the very top of the Eiffel Tower. The guard was nowhere in sight, and the last of the other visitors, disappointed at the overcast view, were shuffling out.

Marcel Brioche leaned over the rail once more and looked down at Paris. To others this might be a breathtaking view, but to Brioche it was merely a good place to jump. He had run over all the excuses for living; none seemed to apply in his case. Life without *her* was worthless. If it were not that his country needed him now, if it were not too selfish an act, he could simply grip this rail in both hands and...

"I beg your pardon, maybe you don't remember me," said a voice in English. He turned to regard a tall, thin young man in a green eyeshade and a trenchcoat. A press card stood in the band of the eyeshade.

"I'm very sorry," said the astronaut. "I have no wish to make a statement at this time ... perhaps later..."

"Don't you remember me? In Marrakech? I'm Beele of the CIA," Beele growled hoarsely.

Brioche's manner chilled. "I'm afraid I have nothing to say to you at any time," he said. "I suppose it was you who knocked me unconscious in that alley?"

"No, it was *you* who slugged *me*."

"And now you want revenge?"

"No, I'm authorized by my government to offer you a substantial emolument, pursuant to only the most minor of conditions."

"A bribe, eh?" The astronaut grinned. "I knew it would come to this. I see your government has not yet stopped trying to buy honour—in which, therefore, it must still be deficient. I am not so poor, however, that I need to sell my country."

"I'm not asking you to sell your country. Just stop making speeches and accusations against the US. It's only a matter of easing international tensions ..."

Brioche lit a cigarette. "Easing up on pressure where more should be applied, you mean. Tell me, can you look me in the eye and say there is no American agent aboard our ship? Eh?"

Avoiding his eye, Beele said, "I'm prepared to offer a million francs. Think it over. A million! Look at that glittering city out there, and think how far a million would carry you."

"I live as well as many millionaires now, and I have my good conscience," said the Frenchman. "There is only one thing I wish —to bring someone dead back to life again—and that cannot be done, not with a million worlds of money."

"You mean the girl you told me about? Listen, I'm sorry about that. Tell you what. How would you like to meet a new girl—like *this* girl, for instance?" Barthemo Beele dug out his billfold and extracted a mildewed snapshot of Mary Junes Beele. "Not bad, eh?"

The astronaut tried to shove it away, but his eyes lingered on it just a second too long. "Yes," he admitted. "I would like to meet her."

"Nothing could be easier. Uh, we haven't been in touch lately, but the government could dig her up for you in a day or so. Now—"

"I meant to say, I would like to meet her under any other circumstances but these. Hers is the first face I have seen that might help me forget the face of another.

"But I know, alas, you are trying to *sell* me this woman. And not only could I never accept any favours from you or your government, but it saddens and troubles me to think what you are doing to her. I know the girl who owns this face could never let herself be used so insidiously. It is only with the greatest difficulty that I prevent myself from treating your base suggestion with the contempt it so richly deserves."

"Listen, I'm sorry. I didn't realize—crude of me, wasn't it? No hard feelings, I hope. No offence intended—"

The astronaut turned away and gazed at the overcast sky. "You don't understand," he said, "what *she* meant to me. If not for duty's sake, I would kill myself."

"Why not?" Beele said, changing pace smoothly. "Why not just throw yourself over the side now? What do you really have to live for? A political career? A few honours and a movie of your life? What do these mean?"

"No!" The astronaut's voice trembled.

"But what a magnificently romantic gesture. At the height of your glory, with every woman in the republic swooning over you, you kill yourself for a broken heart! All you have to do is just grasp the rail in both hands and throw yourself—"

"No! My country needs me! My people—"

"Do they? Aren't you just as much a hero to them dead as alive? Might you not be even more useful dead?"

"No! I reject all three of your repugnant offers. Begone! Goodbye!"

Suddenly Beele was trembling with fury. What right did this guy have to order him around? Didn't he know Beele could kill him at any time? There had clearly been no point in delaying the special treatment this long.

"Goodbye, is it? What do you mean, goodbye? Are you thumbing your nose at the United States Government's more-than-generous offer? Are you even refusing to sleep with my wife? I used to think you were a decent guy—I even told Suggs as much—but now I see he was right! Goodbye it is, then—you dirty F-f-f—" For the first time in his life, Beele found himself stuttering. He tried again, but the word refused to come. The astronaut waited patiently, not coaching, not laughing, merely standing by, and somehow this very patience infuriated Beele all the more, and aggravated his stutter. Finally he gave up, and flung himself at his victim without benefit of a final insult.

The CIA's excellent manual of combat techniques was brief but thorough, and Beele had memorized every word of it. Assuming the stance of the crudely-printed little figure on page 42, he seized the Opponent's arm and twisted it from A to position B. Then he kicked out with his (burning) left foot while pivoting on the bunion of his right. Placing heel of left foot under Opponent's armpit, as on page 43, he levered Brioche into space.

"Look, the Eiffel Tower!" Ron shouted. "Hey, Mac, like in *Zazie*. Let's go up to the top, what say?"

Kevin Mackintosh snapped his fingers. "Yeah, and then get even higher."

"Shouldn't you be up at the top, making sure people don't jump off?" Mary asked the guard.

He laughed. "No one ever jumps off the Eiffel Tower. And the only ones up there now are Marcel Brioche and some reporter. They wouldn't have any reason for jumping, especially not The Astronaut."

She clicked her cough drop thoughtfully. "He might," she said. "Say, if he had a secretly-broken heart. Or someone could push him off."

"They say that the specially-tailored space suit he wears has a built-in parachute. But come, my little, let us talk of other things. Have you ever seen a Paris bachelor's apartment?"

"Dozens," said Mary, sighing with fatigue and boredom. "And they're all the same. Like their occupants." She thought of the sameness of the men in her past: Harry (good old Harry Stropp! Hooves on the roof! As she remembered him he would always be skipping rope and grinning), Cal, Barty (with his worn, too-clever prose, reminiscent of the early *Time* magazine: "Backward ran sentences until reeled the mind."), the sailor with the tattooed arms, the technical writer (author of *The Fork Lift Truck*, as he never tired of telling people), the industrialist who had brought her to Paris...

They were depressingly the same, even to this guard. No, she knew there was only one man who could ever mean more to her

158

than free cough drops—the man now at the top of the tower—Marcel Brioche. Yesterday she had stood in the rain three hours listening to him speak, even though she could not understand his language. Today she had heard he was going up in the Eiffel Tower, and she had started up the stairs to the top, half-intending to throw herself in his way. But for the first time in her life a strange shyness overcame Mary. She dawdled now, half-way up the tower, talking to a guard with whom it was not going to be possible to talk reasonably for very much longer.

"My room is just around the corner—" he said.

"Tell me, what are those little grey boxes running all over the girders?"

"Those? I suppose they are some new inspection or repair machines. I notice they have been replacing many of the old girders with new. But let us talk, rather, of girdles. You American women all wear girdles, I know. Tell me—"

"But what is that big iron drum down there in the centre?" she asked. "It looks like a gas mantle, only hundreds of times larger. And what is all that machinery in the centre? I don't know the Eiffel Tower had all that junk in it."

"I do not know. Who pays any attention to such mundane technical matters, my little? Let us talk rather of—"

There was a faint cry from above.

"Someone has fallen!"

"*Merde*. On my shift. I'd better get down and keep the crowds back."

Mary looked at the body above, hurtling down towards her, a body dressed in a silvery space suit. So he had jumped! She saw it all in a flash—he had jumped for love! Some woman had caused him to despair. As he slid past, his handsome face white and rigid, Mary made a sudden decision.

"Wait for me!" she cried, and leaped after him.

Suddenly he pulled a zipper and a tricolor chute snapped out. She was in his arms.

"You!" he exclaimed. "The woman in the picture! But do you know this Barthemo Beele?"

"I'm married to him," she said. "Temporarily. Gee! How do *you* know him?"

"Why, he's the one who pushed me off! This is indeed my lucky day," he said. "To escape death narrowly and at the same time meet the woman of my dreams—the woman I have waited all my life for—and I owe it all to your husband!"

Tears of happiness stood in his eyes. Mary swallowed her cough drop and kissed him.

Barthemo Beele looked at the dwindling speck with a certain workmanlike sense of accomplishment. He had, after all, successfully given his first special treatment. It was almost like passing an initiation. Suggs would have been proud.

A second tiny figure leapt from the middle of the tower somewhere and joined the first, and almost at the same time a bright parachute blossomed. Was it possible? Was Brioche escaping his special treatment?

"No! It's not fair! I've been cheated! Come back here, you cheating Frog! Come back!"

The tower began to tremble under him. That was all he needed, now. That would make everything perfect, if the damned thing fell down with him. Talk about poetic injustice.

It was only after a minute or two that he realized the Eiffel Tower was not falling—quite the contrary.

"Look, the Eiffel Tower!" Ron shouted. "Like in *Seven Against Mars*, or *It Came In Outer Space*."

"Not again," breathed Kevin.

"A freakout. Man, I can't wait to get to New York and try that with the Empire State building."

CHAPTER XXI

THE PORTEUS EFFECT

"If you were queen of pleasure
And I were king of pain."
SWINBURNE

Dr. Smilax entered the recovery room just as Susie was waking. "How do you feel?" he asked. While taking her pulse, he avoided the girl's gaze.

"Oh Doctor, my throat is so sore!" she whispered.

"That's normal for tonsilectomies," he said shortly. "Yes, yes, we all must suffer."

"But I don't mind." She said it rather doubtfully, and her chin trembled as she squeaked, "I'm so happy?"

He pretended to study her chart minutely.

"You—you haven't lost respect for me, have you?" Her eyes brimmed with tears. She tried to take his hand but he pulled it away.

"Why no, of course not—Susan. I respect you a great deal. Really."

"No, you don't! You hate me! Oh, I knew I should never have given in! I gave you my tonsils and now—now it's 'Susan'!"

As her wail rose in pitch the doctor grew restless—the way a well-mannered dog grows restless when he hears a siren. It was clear that he would rather be elsewhere. Once more, he assured her he felt the deepest respect for her, but his voice had an impatient edge and he spoke looking at the wall.

"No, you don't! You don't care for me at all! You won't even look at me!"

He turned to her as an arachnologist to a specimen long since added to his collection, that had turned out not to be very interesting after all.

"I don't hate you," he said. "It's you who should hate me, and perhaps that is what you meant to say, that you do hate me. I don't blame you, my dear. We should never have met, I see that now. I'm ages too old for you."

"But if we love each other, what does age matter?" she said, sniffling.

He started out the door without answering. Then he paused, without looking back, and said, "I'll order an air ambulance to take you home."

The girl turned her face to the wall.

How odd, Smilax thought, that she who had meant so much to him before the operation now meant no more than a pair of symmetrical tonsils. Seated at his desk, he rolled the bottle in his hand, watching the two spongey objects with a detachment that amazed him. He was even somewhat indifferent to the pleasure to be got out of abandoning her. He just didn't care.

There were so many more important things to care about now. A few hours ago he had come out of surgery expecting to find Aurora Candlewood tormenting an abject Grawk. Instead, there had been no sign of either.

The control booth console told him what had happened: Aurora had released Grawk from his cage, then made her escape through the literal-mindedness of the System. She was by now on her way west, with a .87 probability of stopping at the Wompler Lab and a .11 probability of going on to California.

Smilax typed: "Where is Airman Grawk?"

"ASSUMING AIRMAN GRAWK MEANS THE SAME AS AIRMAN THIRD CLASS GRAWK, HE IS AT COORDINATES 555A31,996B29,201H56, NORAD."

"What is the name of the room he is in?"

"THE NAME OF THE ROOM IS 402 OR LOUNGE."

"What has happened to him?"

"HE ATTEMPTED TO MOLEST DR. CANDLEWOOD. HE WAS SUBDUED BY OPERATION FRIGHTWIG AND IS RESTING QUIETLY IN A SOFABED."

"Is he dead?"

After a pause, during which the System undoubtedly checked to see if Grawk were dead, it reported "NO."

"Imprison him, then, according to Plan Ixion."

That had been hours ago, and still Smilax had not gone to see his prisoner. Ordinarily he would have been glad to spend a few pleasant hours bedevilling him, but today was different. Today a warmth had gone out of Smilax's life—Aurora Candlewood. To-day a chill had crept into it—the Porteus effect.

He was upset that Aurora had left him like this, but what really frightened Toto Smilax was the means by which she had left: *She had tricked the literal-minded Reproductive System.* And if it were possible to trick it once, the trick might be repeated twice, a dozen, a thousand times. The System might be fooled in greater matters, might be cozened into blunders fatal to itself—*or to its creator.*

If there was one thing Smilax feared, it was that someday, somehow, his brain-child would turn on its master and KILL. How many cases there were of this very kind of occurrence, he shuddered to contemplate. Fiction abounded with famous cases like Frankenstein and Rossum('s Universal Robots), with ill-tempered Genii, sorcerers' apprentices and unlucky pacts with the devil. But more horrifying by far was the factual history of the Porteus family, wherein eight generations of geniuses had been murdered by their own devices. Now, whether to frighten or reassure himself he knew not which, Smilax took from the secret drawer of his desk a dusty genealogy and read therein of the Porteus effect.

Passing over the Puritan preacher, Interest Porteus (1680–1720, who, having burned 45 witches, was accidentally hanged on a new scaffold of his own design), he read of Nathaniel Porteus, (1710–63), printer and inventor. Nathaniel had devised a kind of rotary press which automatically turned out the paper twice as fast as his competitors could manage. But one day Nathaniel disappeared:

> The Officers asked var'ous neyghbours had they seen or heard anything suspicious from his establishment, and they said Nought but clanking of the Infernal Presse.

Smilax skipped over Tertiary Porteus (1800–1840), inventor of the steam balloon, to read of Emmet Porteus (1830–1891), the barber who invented an automatic shaving machine. He was found one morning in his shop,

> seated in his chair with a towel about his throat, which had been slashed open. The room reeked of soap, and every receptacle over-flowed. Indeed, the very floor ran in foam, blood-tinct from the copiosity of that dread effusion. Lather all over its fiendish metal body, the machine had rusted fast and could no longer move anything but its jaw. This it creaked open, and in ghastly parody of its master, asked me if the day were hot enough for me.

When Smilax had locked away the genealogy once more, and drunk off a dram of medicinal brandy, he recovered himself enough to descend to the place where his prisoner languished.

163

"Good evening, Airman Grawk," he said cheerily. "Ready for more fun and games?"

The former general had been fitted into a peculiar suit, an adaptation of the "blank tank" in which only his head was free. The rest of him was trussed and counter-trussed with cables running on pulleys and light springs. The sum effect was that, no matter how slightly Grawk moved, he delivered work to the System.

"You will be fed three ounces of chocolate per day," Smilax informed him, "that is, if you do enough work to burn up that much food. On any day your work rate falls below the minimum, your ration will be curtailed. Naturally you will not receive a bonus for exceeding the minimum. Three ounces a day will keep you fit, I should think, for many, many months— perhaps even for years—though your mind will doubtless fail."

"Lemme out of here!" Grawk screamed, flailing his arms in puppet fashion. The spring tensions were so set that he could not bring any part of his body into contact with any other part, nor could he catch hold of the cables. He raged and turned monkey-toy somersaults in vain.

"You just wait," he bellowed. "The US government is going to have plenty to say about this."

"Grawk, you don't seem to understand. There are no United States any more. The United States are a thing of the past."

"What'd you say about my country? Listen, if I wasn't tied up like this—"

"No, *you* listen. I'm going to bring you up to date, Airman Grawk, if for no other reason than that I can see it will make you more miserable."

He switched on a tape of recent radio news coverage:

"In London today, the Society for the Protection of Life on Other Planets held a massive meeting in Trafalgar Square, to welcome, they said, the superior creatures which are taking over our planet. These benevolent creatures, which they refer to as the Galactic Guardians, are allegedly taking over to prevent us from waging a disastrous war.

"Meanwhile, in the rest of the city, thousands of vehicles were caught in an immense traffic jam, caused by both the malfunction of computer-operated traffic lights and the appearance in un-precedented numbers of operating, driverless cars.

"In Paris, the government explained in part the recent ascent into space of the Eiffel Tower. The Space Ministry admitted plotting such an ascent, but claimed it was only a 'theoretical problem for our computers'. They were at a loss to explain how the plan was put into action, but hinted mysteriously at some connection with the collapse of the American Embassy building. The government is resigning today, at the request of the army, which is itself disbanding.

"The Bonn government has capitulated to the newly-formed Dada Party, which has declared its policies to be 'Jam tomorrow and jam yesterday, but never jam today', and 'Every man his own football'.

"In New York, the Brooklyn, Verrazzano and George Washington bridges have been declared unsafe for any traffic, after the removal of iron-work and pilings by what have been described as 'vessels not powered by men'. Following the collapse of several midtown buildings, the island of Manhattan is being evacuated via boats and tunnels.

"The Kremlin has officially declared war on the United States of America, but agreed not to bomb the American continent pending the official resignation of the US Government, which is momentarily expected. There have been reports of missile activity, both US and Russian, but so far no reports of bombings."

Smilax switched off the tape. "There won't be any bombings," he said smugly. "Those US missiles aren't carrying warheads. They're equipped with 'lifting body' capsules, capable of flying in and landing like aircraft, and these are crammed with cells of the Reproductive System—little grey boxes, to you."

"You're lying!" Grawk screamed hoarsely, sawing his arms and legs in the air.

"That's the spirit, Grawk! Give it all you've got!"

Smilax laughed all the way back to his office.

As he settled in the dental chair and began drilling at one of his cuspids, however, the doctor felt his mood change from merriment to melancholy. But why should he be so unhappy? Why did he feel like throwing back his head and howling? Was he not about to be Master of the World?

The answer was obvious: There was no mistress with whom he could share his kingdom. Ah, yes, that was the root of it. Susie was sweet, but—a mere child, a mere entertainment.

But Aurora Candlewood—ah, there was no entremets but a *woman*. Yes, a woman of passions, he was sure, yet also a female scientist, cold as a scalpel blade, impersonal as electricity. He would have given her anything—but she had deserted him.

Suddenly he stopped drilling and leaned forward to spit. Why give up so easily? Faint heart ne'er etc., after all. Thus far he had scarcely made known his feelings to her. Perhaps she did not yet understand the depth of his regard.

He would go after her! He would! He would woo and pursue her until she *had* to say yes.

But if she did not? If she refused? He set the thought aside. There was plenty of time to imagine what he would do if she turned him down. What he would do to himself—and to the world.

CHAPTER XXII

THE BROTHERS FRANKENSTEIN

"Whether or not we could retain some control of the machines, assuming that we would want to, the nature of our activities and aspirations would be changed utterly by the presence on earth of intellectually superior beings."
M. L. MINSKY in *Scientific American*

"I HAVE BECOME more and more certain," Brian Gallopini expostulated, "that this Reproductive System has not only a right to exist, but a duty to thrive; that it is, in many senses, a more legitimate heir to the earth than we. Mark you: it is sturdier, larger, able to reproduce better and quicker than is man. It is as intelligent as man, and certainly quicker of wit. *Enfin*, I can have no doubt but that it is morally incorruptible and just, from what happened to Harry—poetic justice."

Carrying sacks of provisions, the three travellers had just alighted from the grocery van near Millford, Utah, and were now toiling up a great metal ramp into the city.

"And where there is poetic justice, there must needs be a poet to mete it out:

> *Who sees with equal eye, as God of all,*
> *A hero perish or a sparrow fall,*
> *Atoms and systems into ruin hurled,*
> *And now a bubble burst, and now a world.*

"I think this Brobdingnaggian System contains more justice and wisdom than a thousand poets—more than even its makers poured into it," he went on, turning his watery gaze from Daisy to Cal. "And I wonder if our errand here might not be a false one? Could it be that we are sentencing to death a nobler spirit than our own? One more deserving of life?"

Cal cleared his throat. "I'm not at all sure we *can* do anything here," he said. "And I prefer to think we're only shutting off an appliance. It's a temporary measure, after all, till we learn to control the System."

"That's just it," said the Professor. "Is it right for *us* to control

167

it? Might not our petty human ends disgrace and tarnish this most wonderful engine? Might we not pervert it from its true destiny—from Ultimate Harmony with the Universe? It is, after all, a colony of creatures superior in every way."

"It *does* seem superior," Cal admitted, pointing to the Wompler Laboratory, from which issued forth a constant stream of grey boxes. There was not a trace of electric power cabling, smoke, dust or noise. "That, for instance, is my idea of a perfect factory. But shouldn't there be more to superiority than just efficiency? And if we shut it off, are we not proving ourselves its superior in at least ability to survive?"

"Sophistry!" Brian shouted. "It is sinful, yes, *sinful* to tamper with rational perfection. The Reproductive System is the embodiment of all that is right and reasonable. It cannot, it must not be diluted by our vexatious theories. If there is not room for man, so be it! *Let man step aside,* so that his greater, more perfect successor may have room in which to grow!" Shaking out his snuff-stained handkerchief, he blew his nose with a vigorous and angry flourish, then led the way into the Wompler Research building.

"Put up your hands!" shouted a faint, distant voice. "Get over against that wall!" After looking about, they discovered the voice to emanate from a thin, hungry-looking youth in a Marine Corps dress uniform, who sat on the floor at their feet. He seemed to be struggling with something at his side, and at length drew forth a .45 automatic. Slowly, holding it with both hands, he raised the gun to train upon them. It wavered there for a second, then dropped to the floor. The youth made unhappy noises and assumed an unhappy expression. "You shouldn't go in without a pass," he said, again the faint, faraway voice.

"Here." Daisy exchanged the gun for a chocolate cupcake from her sack of groceries. Brian accepted the gun and tucked it away in one of the deep pockets of his coat while Daisy peeled the cupcake for the young man.

"Who are you?" Daisy asked the guard. "What are you doing here, you poor thing?"

"I don't have to tell you anything but my name, rank and serial number," he replied, taking a sullen bite of a second cupcake.

"Are you strong enough to walk, if we help you?" Cal asked.

"I'm staying right here till I'm relieved!"

The marine was adamant. After a consultation, during which

Brian called the boy a "pertinacious puppy", the three divided their provisions into four parts, left one part with him, and moved on down winding corridors, ever more gloomy.

The building seemed utterly deserted. Cal found the door to the cafeteria impossible to budge, and it seemed to be seeping cold, greasy liquid around the edges.

They climbed to the upper level, where the dim hall was lined with rough iron plates. Two parallel grooves had been cut into the floor, for what reason they could not determine.

"This is spooky," Daisy whispered, looking round at the scaly walls. "There isn't a soul anywhere."

"Air," sighed the echo along the length of the hall. Otherwise it was silent, but for an occasional faint drip of water somewhere far in the distance.

"Come on, this way," Cal beckoned. "The laboratory is the last room at the end of the hall, on the right."

"Labra, this, labyrinth, all, right," quavered the liquid echo. It took up their footsteps as they approached the dark end and opened a door.

Bright fluorescent glare streamed across the rust-pitted floor and gleamed in the twin grooves.

"Hello, is anyone here?" Cal shouted.

Pointing a trembling finger to the corner of the room, Daisy said, "Yes and no."

When they stood still, they were so utterly motionless, and when they moved, it was with such blurring speed and precision, that it was impossible to mistake the two armoured figures for humans. They looked alike, with big, square, blocky heads, with cathode-ray tubes where their faces ought to be. They moved about with inhuman agility in utter silence, performing tasks the nature of which Cal could only guess. They wore the red identification badges of Kurt and Karl Mackintosh.

Avoiding the three humans as bats avoid obstacles, they veered gracefully without altering their speed. Now one would carry a smoking test tube to a centrifuge, while the other manipulated a switchboard of test equipment. Now one glided to a typewriter and typed, at blinding speed:

11011 HIGH CTR GRAVITY TIPS GLASS
11012 IRON TOROID KEEPS PROPORTIONS WHILE EXPANDING
11013 THE TRUCK DRIVER IS WRONG
11014 AE2 PLUS BE2 EQUALS CE2

11015 DEFINITION: (DO NOT PUNCTURE OR INCINERATE) MEANS (DO
NOT PUNCTURE) AND (DO NOT BURN) AND (DO NOT PUNCTURE
AND BURN)
11016 OIL FLOATS ON VINEGAR
11017 DOWN IS IN THE DIRECTION OF GRAVITY SOMETIMES
11018 KWALITEIT, HOE WORDT DIE GEMETEN?
11019 HAT: HEAD:: SHOE: FOOT
11020 MILL, JOHN STUART (1806–73): PHILOSOPHER AND ECONOMIST.

At the same time, the other began writing down figures and
equations on a peculiar copper clipboard, using a stylus. Both
stylus and board were connected electrically to the wall.

Now and then one of the two figures would turn to the other
and display upon its face-screen a series of numbers. Otherwise
there seemed to be no conversation between the two, nor any
need for conversation, for they glided about effortlessly in what
seemed almost a ballet of order and harmony. When they finished
a step or process the revolving apertures atop their heads would
swivel towards a display console at the end of the room, but as
soon as it had lighted its WELL DONE sign, the ballet resumed.

"Amazing and beautiful," murmured Prof. Gallopini. "I'd
gladly give up my life of crime to know how such wondrous
engines work."

"I'd give a lot to know how to shut all of this off," Cal mused,
looking around him in some bewilderment. "I don't recognize
any of the equipment I've seen here. If this thing can metamorphose that fast ..."

"Metamorphose? Ah yes," said Brian, looking around with a
smile. "Mere metal transcends itself. These exquisite automa-
tons strive for equilibrium, just as the earth strives to become
a perfect sphere, just as the universe becomes always more
ordered."

"What funny-looking robots!" Daisy remarked. "They have
cast-iron ears! And no mouths!"

"Nor need they mouths," Brian insisted. "These are the men
of tomorrow! These are the inheritors of the earth! These
are the *Übermensch,* the equilibrists, the dynasts!" Extending
his arms towards the busy robots, he declaimed, "Men of the
future, we who are about to become extinct salute thee!"

Without seeming to notice his speech, the two machines carried
out their next task. One opened the lab door, the other lifted
Brian Gallopini and set him on his feet in the hall. Before Cal

170

and Daisy could remark on this, they were given identical treatment.

The hall was far from dark now, and far from quiet. A string of fluorescent tubes along the centre of the ceiling lit up the entire empty length of it, while there was all about a deep rumble, hideous and deafening that made cymbals of the floors and walls. It grew so loud so rapidly that there was not even enough time to ask one another what it meant. Then the far end wall of the corridor split open like a curtain, and the nose of an enormous steam locomotive rumbled towards them.

It moved only at the rate of perhaps one mile per hour, spattering hissing steam as it ground ineluctably towards their cul-de-sac. The brakes were on, and the wheels spewed fire from the grooves as they slid and spun backward, but the engine did not appear to be slowed in the least.

Screaming at one another noiselessly in the din, the three companions pulled at the lab door, their only refuge. It budged open only an inch or two, just enough for Cal to glimpse the two robots pulling it shut. The screen of one displayed a picture of the amused features of Karl; the other showed his twin. Their metal muscles moved, and the door closed against all the efforts of the three humans.

Daisy whirled on Brian and mouthed the words, "Well, get ready for another helping of poetic justice."

The three backed up against the end wall of the corridor, watching Old Number 666 roll towards them.

CHAPTER XXIII

ORBITUARY

"Soon as the evening shades prevail,
The Moon takes up the wondrous tale;
And nightly to the listening Earth
Repeats the story of her birth."

ADDISON

AT TIMES IT seemed to Suggs as if the man across the Monopoly board from him were not Vetch, but someone else. The little Russian's bearded features would gradually blend themselves into those of someone long forgotten, some agent Suggs had killed, or wanted to kill ... but now it was himself Suggs wanted to kill, and the enemy agent who prevented him from doing it.

Suggs had been thinking all day of secret suicide, of killing himself in some way right in front of Vetch by opening a vein inside his suit, or—but it was no use, the Russian caught on too fast. Neither man dared sleep, for fear the other would annihilate himself. Vetch hadn't blinked for hours.

Sleeplessness was affecting Suggs's own mind, he knew, and weightlessness irritated his body. He chafed himself against the straps, or pressed hard against the soft cushion, almost as if to prove his own existence. He felt no more substantial than a spectre.

Haroun Al Raschid took his seat across from him and began talking at once, moving his fat bejewelled hands expressively but making no sound. They were taking a ride on the Reading, Suggs supposed, or the Orient express.

"I'm disoriented," he explained to Haroun. But the fat man went on talking, talking, unaware that his words made no noise, unaware, too, of the purple stain spreading across the front of his pale silk shirt.

Vetch had landed on *Chance*. Had that been the last turn? Suggs found he couldn't remember; he couldn't even remember how many days had gone by since ... since what?

Vetch's face kept changing to that of Scotty, his broken features spattered with blood and bits of bone.

"You really faked me out with that typewriter shotgun, old buddy," he murmured. "It was a good trick, Suggsy."

If he talked to Vetch, he thought, maybe Scotty would go away.

"Have I told you how I killed my first partner in Marrakech?"

"No, I don't believe so. Tell me."

"It was pretty funny. I had this portable typewriter rigged up so the carriage was also a sort of hollow tube that could shoot a shotgun shell. It fired by pressing the question mark."

Scotty spoke, forming sticky bubbles of blood. "The question is, why?"

"He double-crossed me," Suggs said shrilly. "I knew it was him got the other half of that photo of Brioche from Haroun. They were trying to swindle me and sell out to the—to you guys."

"Not to us," said Vetch. "I thought you knew there never was another half to that photo. Brioche's vanity, you see. He never let anyone have a photo of what he called his 'bad side'. I thought you knew that."

"You did know it, Suggsy, but you don't want to remember," Scotty chuckled. "That's the funny part of it. You really just wanted an excuse to kill a couple of people, didn't you?"

"My partner," said Suggs, affecting not to hear him, "would like to weasel out of his death even yet. But I won't let him get away with it. I'm glad I killed him, and if he were alive today, I'd kill him again. I think it must have been him who put her up to it."

"Put who up to what?" asked Vetch.

"Put my wife up to divorcing me."

Laughing, Scotty faded imperceptibly into scowling Vetch. Suggs developed an uncontrollable tremor in his left leg. He thought of his trenchcoat back in Marrakech, and cursed himself for leaving it there. There was cyanide sewn into one epaulet.

Through the tinted faceplate of his helmet, Vetch's savage gaze bored into Suggs's eyes. Vetch did not appear to hear the knock at the door.

The door opened and Barthemo Beele, eyeshade in hand, came in. He had to crouch for the low ceiling, as he moved right over to the chair where Vetch was sitting and sat down *in* him. Grinning self-consciously, he began to crush the brim of the eyeshade.

"I never killed you, at least," Suggs snarled.

"You would have, if you had stayed around long enough, chief," said the earnest young man. He dropped a press card, and it fluttered to the floor.

"That was a mistake, Beele," said Suggs with a nasty laugh. "You forgot there is no gravity here. Things don't fall."

"*I* forgot? If it comes to that, it was *your* mistake," Beele said politely. "Am I a figment of your sleepless imagination or not?"

"I could find out." Suggs reached for his gun, then relaxed and laughed again. "No, you'd like that, wouldn't you? I'd be killing Vetch, which is just what you, my unconscious mind, want me to do."

"Guess again," said Beele, his voice dropping to a whisper. "Vetch has been dead for hours, and you know it."

His smile faded to Vetch's scowl, and the press card in his fingers became an orange *Chance* card. The Russian's face was blue, and there were poison blisters on the lips.

"I'll be damned!" Suggs slapped his knee. "Vetch, you did it, and right in front of me!"

The corpse looked contempt at him. "The question is, what are you going to do?" it said. "You poor son of a bitch."

"I'm gonna radio the news of your death back, and then I'm gonna ... I'm not sure."

He encoded his message and sent it: "IVAN DEAD. FOLLOWING ARE PERFORMANCE TAPES ON EQPT."

There was no need to wait for a reply. He knew what it would order him to do. *Go to hell. Go directly to hell. Do not pass God.* He closed up his suit, hooked in a fresh tank of oxygen, and climbed out of the ship. After straddling it for a moment indecisively, he pushed himself free. At this distance the moon was brighter, but it looked as boringly hieroglyphic to him as ever. He drifted off to sleep, wondering if he were falling away or towards the moon.

He awoke trying to remember if he had finished balancing his bank statement. He did so now, visualizing the neat, meaningful rows of expenditures like a lattice ...

He realized he was looking at a tower, very like the Eiffel Tower, sliding by him slowly. Amazingly real it was. On the top platform he could even make out the tiny, frosty figure of a man, gripping the rail with both hands. For no apparent reason, the man was wearing an eyeshade. Suggs went to sleep.

He awoke trying to remember whether he had finished balancing his bank statement or not. He did so now, wisely deciding not to postpone it. His oxygen was giving out, he supposed; thinking was becoming difficult.

He unsheathed his knife and held it at arm's length. It was a moment to make a fine, self-sacrificing speech, but his oxygen-starved mind was slowing. There was only one speech Suggs could remember:

"Take that, you dirty—!"

The postcards were so banal they just *had* to be code—yet the plain fact was that they weren't. After tearing off the stamps for his nephew's collection, the Russian code clerk consigned Bubby to the incinerator.

CHAPTER XXIV

TIME AND CHANCE

"My mind seems to have become a kind of machine for grinding general laws out of large collections of facts."
DARWIN

CAL FELT A handle on the wall behind him. He twisted it, and a firedoor rolled back smoothly, revealing a new section of hallway. The three companions scrambled into it, the locomotive following at a more dignified pace.

The first door they tried was open. As they ducked into it, Daisy and Cal grinned at one another with relief. Brian's brow remained puckered, however, as he stared at the oncoming engine's wheels and feet.

The wheels were reversing to throw grindstone sparks. Behind the engine, a seemingly endless line of cars creaked and groaned to a halt. Out of the hissing vapour an engineer in goggles descended, pulled off one oily gauntlet, and handed down an attractive young woman.

"Whew!" The engineer whistled. "You people were nearly demised on the spot. That could have been a most unfortuitous vicissitude."

"Dr. Trivian!" Cal shouted, peering at the sand-caked, goggled face. "Is it really you?"

"By gad, it is Calvin Potter!" Trivian seized his hand. "This is indeed an audacious occasion, my boy."

"But what are you doing here? So far from MIT?"

"I am realizing my lifelong dream of driving a steam locomotive. That is, the little grey box does the actual driving, but I am entitled to make suggestions—which are never heeded.

"But I forget myself, or I forget my passenger, which is not the same thing at all, eh? Dr. Aurora Candlewood, may I present my former pupil, Calvin Potter?"

She was nearly Cal's height, slim, with small hands and feet and the shallow breasts and slender, arching neck of a dancer. Yet there was a decided awkwardness about her movements, as if she deliberately chose to disguise her natural grace by holding her body always in stiff, unlovely positions. Her hand was cold.

Cal became depressingly aware of his own uncombed hair, muddy clothes and dirt-grained face. A sudden fiery itch stung his chin where a neophyte beard, tough and patchy, clung desperately as lichen to a crumbling rock. Mechanically he introduced Aurora and Trivian to his companions.

Brian was morose and silent as a watchmaker over Aurora's hand.

"Strangers call me Miss le Duc," said Daisy to the engineer. "My friends call me Daisy. But to remain my friend is to resist the temptation to call me *you know what*."

Aurora explained to them her interest in Project 32 and her purpose in coming to the Wompler Lab. She was relieved at finding in Cal someone who knew something about the functioning of the Reproductive System, from the individual cell level upwards.

Brian announced that he was going to "find out what time it is", and left, by a door leading to a second corridor.

"Yes," said Trivian. "We'll leave you two scientificians to your palaver. Miss le Duc, my arm?" They set off after the gangster.

Aurora and Cal avoided looking at one another as she related to him her adventures with Smilax at NORAD, and told him that the mad dentist was in control of the Reproductive System.

"Smilax in control. Hmm. Wonder how he does it."

Cal defined his own experience with the System, at its inception, in Las Vegas, and on the road back. After mentioning its apparent transmission of acquired characteristics, its occasional abortive mutations, and its manifest kenogenetic tendencies, he added that he thought he loved her.

"I see." She prepared to consider all aspects of the matter gravely. Had he any data on the System's reproduction rate? On its learning limitations, if any? And was it not true that many who thought themselves in love were not?

He told her what he knew about QUIDNAC, and that he hoped to win her hand in marriage.

Aurora, blushing, discussed operant and respondant conditioning, and how the modification of one kind of behaviour might send ripples spreading throughout all of an organism's behaviour, as in the learning of abstract reasoning.

She expressed her hope that the System might be coerced into behaving itself" by (1) establishing rapport; (2) becoming a kind but stern parent to it; (3) channelling the System's functions to humanly useful ends; (4) establishing models of behaviour and a routine of rewards and punishments to guide the System. Of these, (1) would be the hardest.

"If we only knew how Smilax controls the System," Cal said, "we could somehow impersonate him."

"Recognition is a difficult kind of behaviour to analyse," she explained. "Because it goes on, in most people, at the edge of consciousness. We recognize a friend seen in different light, at odd angles, at a distance, or with an added moustache."

"Or aged for fattened, yes. But the literal-minded System can't possibly cope with all that. I'm inclined to think that Smilax uses some kind of badge or password identification—something unique."

Aurora was not so sure. "It wouldn't do to have some cue-object that anyone else might get hold of, or that might be lost. I tend to believe it's something more positive, like fingerprints, ear configurations, retinal pattern."

She added that she would consider his offer of marriage and that she would rather answer later.

Cal was about to point out that there might not *be* a later, when from far away, Daisy screamed.

"Stay here," Cal commanded, and ran from the room.

At some point, Elwood Trivian had taken a wrong turn. One moment he had been walking arm-in-arm with Daisy; they had unlinked arms to pass on opposite sides of a pillar; the next moment he was utterly alone.

Alone, moreover, at the intersection of two empty corridors, down each of which he could see for hundreds of yards. He could not decide which to choose. After a moment's hesitation, he headed to the left.

The floor suddenly wasn't there. Clawing the air, Elwood fell in darkness, trying to remember a childhood prayer: "Bless—"

He struck the water and plunged under, holding his breath. Only it was *not* water, but something greasy and bitter. He broke the surface and took air.

What kind of nightmare was this, anyway? He seemed to be floating in a lake of cold, greenish, slightly viscid coffee. There was light, from somewhere, and there was a ceiling perhaps five feet overhead. Otherwise nothing, in all directions, but choppy

178

waves. He began to tread coffee and bob along like a cigarette butt.

Brian waved a .45 at Cal and Daisy. His dust-coloured, wispy hair was rumpled, and there was a strange, sly look in his eye. He crouched in the centre of the room, next to a metal cabinet.

"Keep back, both of you. This does not concern you."

"What does not concern us?" Cal asked. "What's wrong, professor?"

"Nothing is wrong. On the contrary, everything is right! The time ... the auspices..." He gestured at the metal cabinet, from which, at regular intervals, a foot or two of paper was vomited forth. "And behold the Clock of Life!" He looked up.

Now Cal saw that the ceiling of this round room was a great clock face, perhaps fifty feet in diameter. The minute hand was visibly moving to join the hour hand at twelve, while a red second hand swept out its sectors silently. Daisy cowered against the wall under XII, and now Cal edged towards her from the doorway at III.

Seeing the movement, Brian whirled and fired. Plaster puffed from the wall a few inches from Cal's head.

"I said stay put! Nothing must move—but the clock." He looked up at it and smiled. "Geared to the perfect clockwork of our universe ... set in motion once, for Æternity!" He mumbled something indistinct, then:

"Time flies, you see ... on the pinions of clocks ... time is money, you pays your money and you takes your chance ... round and round she goes, and where she stops ... yes, time must have a stop ... time and chance happen to them all..."

"O God! It's his old illness," said Daisy, turning away. "Games of chance, clocks, magic squares—it's been coming over him for years. I thought if I could get him away from the university, from eighteenth-century clockwork thought, he would be all right. But I suppose the disappointment in Las Vegas, followed by Harry's death, has upset the balance of his mind..."

Brian laughed harshly. "What do any of you know of *balance*? Or of escapement? Or of—"

"Brian, listen to me! It's Daisy! Don't you know me?"

A deafening chime began to announce the hour. A panel in the floor slid open near Brian. He paused only for a second, then leaped into it.

Daisy screamed. Then, though Cal tried to head her off, she ran to the edge of the hole and peered down into it.

What followed could only have been a kind of malevolence on the part of the machine, for now the red second hand began lowering itself as it continued to sweep around, so that it angled down directly towards Daisy's head. She seemed too horrified at what she saw to notice.

Rushing towards her, Cal called, "Daisy, duck!"

"What did you call me?" She turned to give him an indignant look, as the giant second hand caught her alongside the head. She pitched over the edge, and was gone.

Cal ran up to the now-closing panel and looked down. He could see nothing but myriads of gears of all sizes, running smoothly and quietly, Some were stained red.

Elwood Trivian dozed, still treading coffee, and dreamed of his steam engine. The Las Vegas Express kept somehow turning into a Las Vegas expresso machine, and he could not get one steam-chuffing box separated from another...

When he awoke, two men were hauling him out of the lake on to their raft of cafeteria tables. One man was so gluttonously fat and the other so starvelling thin that they seemed almost a part of his dream. Only the smell of coffee reminded him that this was horrible reality.

"Gee, Pop," said the fat man. "He looks hungry." He busied himself about the pages of a magazine. The thin man appeared to take no notice of anything but his immediate task; paddling his feet off one end of the raft to propel it through the coffee.

"Here, fella, eat up hearty," said the fat one, tearing out a picture of roast beef and handing it to Elwood. "There's plenty more where that came from." The engineer sat with it in his hand, dazedly watching fatso devour pictures of cakes and pies.

"Coffee?" He dipped up a dirty paper cup of the sludge near the paddling feet and offered it. Elwood shook his head. "I know whatcha mean. Coffee makes ya so nervous ya can't eat right. I stick with *solid* food."

Pulped-up magazine pages drooled down his slowly-working chin.

The room in which Aurora waited seemed to be a storeroom. Weapons and electronic equipment lay along the walls. There was furniture, a roll-top desk in one corner and a grandfather

180

clock opposite the door. Aurora watched it, as a distant, larger clock began to chime. In a few seconds, the grandfather clock whirred and took up tinny notes of its own. *One, two . . .*

The grandfather clock at home had never run, despite all her father's attempts to fix it. It was not running the day he died.

The inquest found accidental death, resulting from a malfunction of one of his projects, a diving bell. She strove to become tough-minded about his memory. After all, this was a world where clocks ran and trains ran and people ran to catch them. Not a world for losers, whether they were middle-aged farmer-dreamers or young, idealistic lab assistants, like Cal.

Of course Cal was a loser. He was the kind of man, she knew, who ends up at forty running a bankrupt gas station too far from the turnpike. Who, just before he declares bankruptcy, is shot by a feeble-minded bandit for $2.12 in the till. There was probably nothing that Cal could do right.

She thought it more than likely that she would marry him.

. . . eleven, twelve.

The case of the grandfather clock opened like a sarcophagus. Dr. Smilax stepped forth and took her in his arms. Aurora screamed.

CHAPTER XXV

THE RIVALS

"Brothers and Sisters, I bid you beware
Of giving your heart to a dog to tear"

KIPLING

"DON'T SCREAM, MY dear," panted Smilax, as Aurora struggled free. "I mean you no harm. I esteem you, in fact, over all other women in this, my world."

"You must be joking." She edged towards the door.

He blocked her path. "Ah, could I joke about your heart? I would rather throw myself under the wheels of a car," he whined. Seizing her hand, he began to kiss it eagerly. "I want to be your—your best friend. I'll dog your footsteps till you say yes. Dear Dr. Candlewood, be mine—and the world will be yours!"

Disgusted, she freed her hand and turned away. Smilax seized her wrist and flung her about to face him again. "Must I hound you?" he barked. "Must I beg and threaten? Speak to me! Speak!"

As she said nothing, he went on, curling his lip to show sharpened, glittering teeth. "I warn you, if you refuse me, I will not merely kill myself. Oh no, that would be too easy. I would take the *world* with me, and in the most *painful* way possible. And *your* death, my precious, would be the most lingering, most excruciating death of all."

A mournful, pleading look came into the eyes behind the polished lenses. Smilax began to fawn and stroke her arm.

"Is it my age? But I'm frisky, yet, my mistress. Yes, and more than willing to learn new tricks. And you could not find, in all the younger men of this world, a more faithful and constant friend than Toto.

"It amused me to hear you and Potter trying to guess how the System 'knows' me—you will *never* learn that secret. But I was less amused to hear that impudent puppy offer you marriage!

"You must choose between us. You must choose between the kindest, truest, richest possible friend, and that ungrateful, ill-bred cur, Calvin Potter."

He caught up both her wrists. "Choose now!"

"Take your filthy paws off her!"

Without waiting for the doctor to comply, Cal lunged at him, throwing an awkward punch. The wily surgeon twisted, so that the blow glanced off his ear and caught Aurora on the side of the face. Her head snapped back against the metal wall and she folded gracefully to the floor.

"Aurora!" both men yelped, diving to help her up. The corner of Smilax's cheek caught Cal in the eye. They began to wrestle, Smilax shoving Cal towards the open panel of the clock.

Suddenly Cal was seized from behind in an iron grip. A stunning blow at the nape of his neck blurred his vision. Something hit him in the kidney, in the stomach, across the bridge of his nose. There seemed to be four, six, a dozen fists pummelling him from all directions. He hit out blindly, encountering no one. It came almost as a relief when something hit him hard in the Adam's apple, and as the grip relaxed he sank into soft darkness.

But he was out only for a few seconds. When he came to, Smilax and two other figures were standing over him. Cal's dazed vision travelled up from wheeled feet and steel legs to armoured bodies and finally to impassive cathode-ray tubes where faces ought to be.

"Ah, you're awake, so the fun can begin. 'Kurt' and 'Karl' here are going to torture you to death—crudely, of course, for they've never done it before—but with the painstaking slowness only machines can manage." Smilax opened the roll top of the desk in the corner to reveal a console. As he pressed a switch on the console, a pedestal chair seemed to sprout from the floor like a mushroom. Smilax settled into it with a sigh.

"Let me see now," he said, brooding over the console. "Nothing serious until Aurora wakes up to watch. I wouldn't want her to miss the main feature, eh? Now, how about starting off with—"

He lifted a doll attached to the console by a thick cable and began massaging its scalp with ungentle vigour. "A dutch rub!"

The two robots dragged Cal to his feet, and while one held him the other performed the same operation. Cal began to yell.

"Ha ha, very good. Now we'll give you an Indian burn, and then twist your arm until you holler uncle." Smilax demonstrated with the doll, and the robots zealously followed suit.

Cal found each torture every bit as painful as he remembered it from childhood. He was beginning to form a plan of escape from his mechanical torturers, but thinking became increasingly difficult as he was given hits and no returns, as his head was thumped and his ears boxed, his toes stepped on and his hair pulled. When not otherwise occupied, the robots were under standing orders to pinch him, which they did in an orderly manner. He noticed they did not both receive their orders from Smilax directly. Only the one wearing Karl's badge would turn the sensing device atop its head to watch Smilax. Then it would light a series of numbers on its face, which "Kurt" would duly note and obey. Cal decided to interrupt their communication.

He waited until Aurora groaned as if coming to her senses. The doctor looked around at the sound, and Cal rammed his elbow into "Karl"'s cathode-ray tube face hard. The implosion drove the robot back a few steps, but it did not lose its balance. It seemed to pause for a second, making up its mind about some electronic matter.

Then "Karl" charged—and began trying to twist "Kurt"'s arm. "Kurt" let go of Cal to fend off its brother. The two began to shuffle, locked in alternating hammer-locks, turning slowly about the room.

Seeing what had happened, Smilax snatched up a rifle-like instrument and pressed it to Aurora's head. "Come near me and she gets it," he snarled.

"Cowardly cur!"

"I'll make you pay for that remark, Potter. Every dog will have his day, and rest assured this will be mine." He pointed the rifle at Cal and fired. A tiny rocket streaked forth, slamming into the wall near him. Cal threw himself at the doctor and seized the rifle before he could fire again. They struggled.

"Kurt! Karl! Help!" Smilax cried.

But the unfortunate robots were of no use. They were still putting hammer-locks on one another, and at that moment the two of them disintegrated, collapsing into fragments which still carried on the combat like the severed claws of crabs.

Cal and the doctor both gripped the launcher-rifle, battering at each other clumsily. They were far from expert fighters, and Smilax's middle age was well-matched by Cal's weary flabbiness. They stumbled over a pair of metal arms which seemed to be Indian wrestling on the floor. Cal lost his balance, then regained it, but by that time the doctor had levered him up against the wall, the launcher across his throat like a quarterstaff.

184

"I should have killed you when I had the chance," Smilax growled, baring his teeth in a grimace.

Cal shoved him back and grinned. "It's you who'll play dead dog Toto!"

"Die!" snapped Smilax, accompanying this with another shove.

"After you!" retorted Cal, shoving him back.

They continued to shove one another and trade insults in one corner of the room. In a second corner, Aurora still lay unconscious. Elsewhere lay scattered robotic parts, including the severed head of "Kurt", whose face displayed only rows of neatly-spaced stars.

"Down, boy!"

Giving one final shove, Cal flung the doctor free of the weapon, then aimed it at him.

"All right!" Smilax screamed. "All right! Go ahead! Shoot me!"

Cal threw down the weapon. "I don't need this," he said, "to bring you to heel."

Laughing, Smilax scooped up the severed leg of a robot and pitched it at him. It caught Cal across the forehead, and he fell backwards into a pile of junk. He was only dimly aware of the doctor's fumbling a pistol from a drawer of the desk. A shot rang out. Cal hit the floor. He looked up in time to see the tail of Smilax's white coat disappear around the edge of the doorway. Cal jumped to his feet and ran after him. Sprinting into the hall, he found himself in a labyrinth of unmarked passages.

The architecture in this part of the building seemed not to be a fixed structure, but a kind of dynamic principle. Varying according to some obscure formula of its own, it altered shapes and sizes constantly. Walls advanced, turned, retreated or collapsed, ceilings buckled and bulged, floors tilted alarmingly or dropped away like elevators. A door might lead to a room fifty stories high, or to one only an inch deep, or it might be false.

One pair of identical rooms contained a window between them, so that, gazing from one monotony of office furniture to the next, Cal wondered for a second at this curious mirror that failed to reflect him. He hurried out, and as he stepped over the threshold, the room behind him collapsed like a card castle.

As he stepped on it, a stairway might become a floor, a ramp, or an escalator. At any time an entire room might be given a quarter turn, might be tilted on its side, might shrink or swell to some new shape. Stairways became floors, ramps, escalators; they led to closets or twisted back upon themselves. From time to time Cal glimpsed the white-coated figure of the doctor; the gap between them was not closing. They made their way upward.

Cal passed through a final trapdoor to the roof, and there was nothing more above but the star-pierced firmament. The roof resembled nothing so much as a giant parking lot of perhaps a hundred acres, with here and there the dim yellow glow from a string of jury-rigged lights. In place of cars there were regularly-spaced, bulky stacks of lumber and crated machinery, covered with canvas. Cal could see, in the distance, fork lifts moving to and fro. Otherwise, nothing moved. There was no sign of Smilax.

Cal crept from shadow to shadow until he reached the edge of the roof. Curious, he peered over—and froze. There were trucks and tanks moving down there. He could obscure the largest ones with the ball of his thumb. It was at least fifty stories to the ground.

A shot rang out and Cal threw himself flat, then began crawling rapidly towards one of the stacks of lumber.

All at once an engine started up somewhere near at hand. A spotlight came on, picking out Smilax crouching on top of a pile of crates. The surgeon threw up one hand to protect his eyes. Another spotlight came on. Under the roar of the motor, Cal could hear a number of voices in excited argument. After a moment the second light went off again. Smilax stood as if transfixed by the single beam, the gun hanging limp in his hand.

A shadow passed overhead and Cal looked up. A crane boom was swinging towards Smilax. The doctor saw it too, and began to whimper. "It is the Porteus effect! The System has gone berserk! It's going to turn on its master, just as I knew it would!" The boom slowed, but kept coming. "Help!" Smilax begged. "Master, don't punish me!"

The boom stopped, and started moving away, and Smilax suddenly took courage.

"Go ahead, try to kill me!" he screamed, jumping up and down and shaking his fist. "I defy you, you nut-and-bolt nightmare! *I'm* the master here, even Potter and Aurora know that. I alone can control you—with these!" He tore off his rimless glasses and waved them aloft. They shone in the harsh light. The strangely-shadowed, naked face of Smilax bared its teeth and growled.

The crane boom moved in his direction once again, and now its clamshell lowered towards him like a giant, cruel jaw. Smilax shrieked and scampered down off the pile of packing cases, and, just as if it had not realized this, the clamshell seized the pile and lifted it.

"Haha, did you think you had me? You filthy, clumsy monster, you missed! All right, go ahead and turn on your creator! If I cannot control you no one shall—ever!" He flung down the glasses and crushed them under his heel.

"Hahaha! Down with the System! Down with the machine!" he bayed, and began to caper in a circle, almost like a puppy chasing its tail. "To hell with cats! Down with Albert Payson Terhune! Screw Lassie! Piss on lamp-posts!"

The pile of boxes fell, suddenly, barely missing him, and there was a splintering crash and the clamshell came down on top of them. Smilax leapt away and turned to bark furiously at the wreckage. The tarpaulin stirred slightly, and from the shadows under it came an ominous clicking. It was as the sound of many knitting needles knitting many dog sweaters—or dog shrouds.

Cal shivered.

"No! No!" shrieked Smilax. "Good boy. Down. Nice System."

The spotlight followed him as he backed away towards the edge of the roof. "No! No! Stay away!" he called, throwing one leg over the railing. "Stay away from me!" But the clicking sound seemed to leave the wreckage and move through the darkness after him, and now it was accompanied by a faint, quavering murmur, high-pitched and eerie.

"Stay away!" he screamed one last time, then threw himself over the edge. Cal rushed to the rail and looked down. He could see nothing of Smilax, but hear his faint scream: "Bowowowow-owowowow!"

The spotlight remained fixed on the splice where he'd gone over. Into its beam a moment later, clicking ominously, marched a swarm of little girls in red-white-and-blue spangles. Mewing as they toddled, two gross of Wompler's Walking Babies followed Smilax over the edge.

The motor of the crane died. The spotlight swung round to pick out the driver, Aurora. She was wearing glasses.

"Are you all right?" she and Cal shouted at the same time.

She climbed down from the cab and ran towards him. Cal ran towards her.

"Get that goddamned spotlight out!" shouted an argumentative voice.

"But, Pop, no one can see if—"

"I don't want any ifs. We got to economize somewhere. Out!"

Stumbling along in the darkness, Cal and Aurora ran on towards one another.

CHAPTER XXVI

UTOPIA

*"The good ended happily, and the bad unhappily.
That is what Fiction means."*

WILDE

CAL AND AURORA were in New York, some weeks later,
holding hands in front of a QUIDNAC machine.

"DEARLY BELOVED," it typed. "WE ARE GATHERED HERE TODAY ..."

Much had happened since the death of Smilax. The dragon was
slain, the frog turned into a prince, and the pudding got off the
end of the nose. Or that was the way Grandison Wompler, the
new President of the United States, spoke of it. In any case, the
Reproductive System had become, under the guidance of Cal and
Aurora, a friend to man.

Cal had asked his fiancée how it was she'd guessed the secret
of Smilax's glasses—in the nick of time.

"I had plenty of time to think, while I was lying there, playing
unconscious," she said. "So I tried to combine our two theories.
You thought the cue must be some sort of talisman, while I
was sure it was something personal and idiosyncratic. The only
thing that fitted both theories had to be that pair of rimless
glasses. I suppose the System had some way or another of testing
them by shooting light through them.

"When you two left, I looked all over for a spare pair. Then it
occurred to me, he wouldn't dare keep a spare pair around, lest
someone should get them. At the same time, he'd have to have
access to another pair, because otherwise he'd have to stop being
God while he went to an optician. So I asked the System to make
me a duplicate pair to his prescription, and it did, in seconds.
Then I was God. I took the elevator to the roof, where I met the
Womplers and Elwood Trivian and so on."

The System had made considerable changes in the political look
of things. Upon his election, Grandison Wompler had embarked
on a speaking tour of the Russian provinces, speaking chiefly
before ladies' clubs. At the same time, the new Premier of the
Soviet Union had engaged to speak to the ladies of Nebraska and

Iowa. These were not cultural exchange programmes, but the main duties of the heads of state now. After all, they had no more paperwork to do—ever. The System had taken care of that.

In fact it had taken over all the jobs no one wanted to do. The System collected garbage and turned it into valuable chemicals like pearls and perfume and maple sugar and fingerpaints.

It did all the dishes in all the homes of the world. It filed all the papers no one wanted to read, and it read them, too. It took care of other distasteful jobs like typing, and like preventing war.

All the typists and government clerks had at first been unhappy about their unemployment. They had, in fact, marched in protest on the System Central in Washington. But the Reproductive System knew very well these women didn't want to break their nails every day on typewriter keys; it found them husbands. It knew these men didn't want to sit around in offices growing lardy-assed and fluorescent-pale; it gave them service medals of pure gold, which they were able to pawn for trips to Mexico.

But perhaps more important even than the happiness of former government clerks was the prevention of war. And this was accomplished by Project LULU (Longrange Unilateral Locking Up). It would lock up, say, a warhead or tank or flamethrower from each nation. Then it would weld up the locks. Then it would pour concrete over the whole thing. Then it would apply very expensive armour plate to this giant block of concrete. Then, if the taxpayers had not tired of the whole mess, it would build sleek, extravagant atom-powered ships for the sole purpose of transporting these big blocks of concrete-preserved armament to a certain rendezvous point in the ocean, where both the U.S. and U.S.S.R. War Rafts were tethered. Each piece of armament was there attached to its nation's War Raft by a long steel cable and lowered to the ocean floor. Thus the two nations were able to build enormous stockpiles of weaponry of the most frightening kind (enough to give their citizens a comfortable glow of security, as frightening weapons always do), but neither could pull a sneak attack. And it was always reassuring to learn that we had faster jets, or a newer kind of bomb, or twice as many bazookas at the bottom as they did.

But someone had to guard our commitment in mid-ocean, so anyone who wished to remain in the military was asked to do his bit of guard duty on our War Raft. Of course there were a number of unpleasantnesses that made War Raft duty less than glorious. First, the American and Russian War Rafts were only a few hundred feet apart, and their occupants were entitled to fire on one another with small arms whenever they liked. Second, food consisted of fried canned peas and powdered eggs in abundance. Seasickness pills were not allotted to the troops. The minimum enlistment was five years, the minimum reenlistment ten years. Finally, the commander of the American Raft was an almost legendary tyrant, one Jupiter Grawk, while the Russian Raft was under the command of a very old, very wicked woman, Gen. Lotte Smilax.

Yes, the System had taken on enough distasteful duties, so that now it was given the very pleasant one of marrying a hero to a heroine.

"DO YOU, CALVIN, TAKE AURORA TO BE YOUR LAWFULLY WEDDED WIFE . . . ?"

With shaking hands, Cal typed, "I do."

"I do," said Jim Porteus, grinning at Susie, his bride. She smiled back, with tears in her eyes. To think that he still cared for her, that he would marry her *now*, even knowing about her tonsils and everything . . . Susie wanted to swoon away with happiness.

Jim Porteus was not really thinking about his marriage at all. He'd thought he might as well get married; that damned machine had taken all the fun out of business and politics. He might as well turn engineer or inventor. Just now he was having an idea for an invention, in fact, that had to make him a fortune. He would call it the "Porteus Automatic Valet," a dignified name for an elegant machine. It would tie one's necktie—any knot wished, just press the button . . .

The minister cleared his throat. "And so you, Susie . . . ?" There was scarcely, he saw, a dry eye in the little chapel at Santa Filomena this morning. A gratifying sight. But there was no one weeping more copiously than poor Madge Suggs. He would have to comfort her, after the ceremony, the minister thought. He would tell her not to think of it as losing a daughter, but as . . .

"I do," said Mary Junes Beele Brioche, in Las Vegas (Nuevas), at the Church of the Psychedelic Saviour.

"Then I now prounce you," intoned His Sacred High Worship, The Very Venerable Kevin Mackintosh, "—or *pronounce* you—astronaut and wife." He began the countdown.

Cal and Aurora had already received tons of cards and telegrams and letters of congratulations, which the System was sorting for them and inserting into the ceremony itself. Now it presented the warmest regards of Elwood Trivian, Ph.D., who announced also the opening of his new School for Steam Locomotive Engineers in Miami (above the dry cleaner's).

Another telegram read:

"MILLFORD, UTAH 10 35 AM. NOT DEAD OF SNAKEBITE AFTER ALL. HAVE BEEN IN SUSPENDED ANIMATION OR SOMETHING FOR PAST SIX WEEKS. CONGRATULATIONS TO I HOPE HAPPY COUPLE. MY HEALTH FINE BUT FOR HOARSENESS FROM EXCESSIVE DICTATION POST-TRANCE. HAVE YOU ANY IDEA WHAT A SIX-WEEKS' TRAIN OF UNBROKEN THOUGHT CAN BE LIKE QUERY. I HAVE INVENTED A NEW ECONOMIC CALCULUS AND HAD A FEW INTERESTING IDEAS ABOUT TRAVELLING FASTER THAN LIGHT. BELIEVE ME, SUSP. ANIMATION IS GOING TO BE THE NEXT DRUG KICK.

"HITA.

"P.S. TELL LOUIE HE IS OFFICIALLY BLACK SCISSORS."

Having delivered this telegram, the QUIDNAC waited until its contents were digested and then typed cautiously:

"I NOW PRONOUNCE YOU MAN AND WIFE, UNLESS YOU HAVE MADE ANY FALSE STATEMENTS IN YOUR APPLICATIONS."

A chute opened and dispensed to them a bag of gold and the ownership of a milkwhite palfrey which awaited them outside, the gifts of a grateful populace.

Cal could not ride, but he helped Aurora up on the horse and led it down Fifth Avenue. All the bells of the city of New York pealed out the glad tidings, while from the office buildings there were released bright-coloured balloons and flocks of snowy doves.

At the Battery, they boarded a barque for a distant land, while all the citizens of New York wept and munched candy and cheered and held up babies to look at them. But for three old men in faded uniforms, who did not look up from their game of Go to the Dump, there was no one in the crowd who did not wish Cal and Aurora happiness, as the barque's white sails filled with wind and it slid silently away from the pier and out to sea.

No. 1   KURT VONNEGUT

The Sirens of Titan

"A classic, ripe with wit and eloquence and a
cascade of inventiveness" – Brian Aldiss
0 575 03819 5

.

No. 2   THEODORE STURGEON

More Than Human

Winner of the International Fantasy Award
"A masterpiece" – James Blish
0 575 03821 7

No. 3   ROBERT SILVERBERG

A Time of Changes

Winner of the Nebula Award
"Highly recommended" – *TLS*
0 575 03820 9

No. 4   SAMUEL R. DELANY

Nova

"His rampaging talent mesmerises the reader" –
Tribune
0 575 03818 7

No. 5   ARTHUR C. CLARKE

The City and the Stars

"One of the most imaginative novels of the
very far future ever written" – *Sunday Times*
0 575 03849 7

No. 6   ROBERT A. HEINLEIN

The Door into Summer

"Highly readable" – *Punch*
0 575 03850 0

No. 7   FREDERIK POHL &
C. M. KORNBLUTH

Wolfbane

"A work of sheer, exuberant imagination" –
Arthur C. Clarke
0 575 03852 7

No. 8   JOHN SLADEK

The Reproductive System

"Superb entertainment . . . full of invention, wit
and subtly sad comedy" – *Sunday Times*
0 575 03851 9

All at £2.95